My Accidental Diet

Wellness and Weight Loss
A New Side of Food and Fitness

Rhonda J Fransoo

eat · breathe · grow

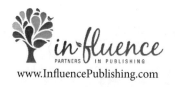

www.InfluencePublishing.com

Published by Eat Breathe Grow, October, 2018
ISBN: 9781999451806

Editors: Rhonda Fransoo and Liane McLaren
Typeset: Greg Salisbury
Proofreader: Lee Robinson
Book Cover Design: Judith Mazari
Book Cover Photo: Bailey Marshall

DISCLAIMER: The information provided in this book is designed to provide helpful information on the subjects discussed. This book is not meant to be used, nor should it be used, to diagnose or treat any medical condition. For diagnosis or treatment of any medical problem, consult your own physician. The publisher and author are not responsible for any specific health or allergy needs that may require medical supervision and are not liable for any damages or negative consequences from any treatment, action, application or preparation, to any person reading or following the information in this book. References are provided for informational purposes only and do not constitute endorsement of any websites or other sources. Readers should be aware that the websites listed in this book may change.

This book is dedicated to my husband and my son
for supporting and encouraging me to fulfill my
life-long dream of writing a book. Also to the Angel
who whispered in my ear that summer day:
"If you write it, you will be supported."

Wishing you
health and wellness
always.
Rhonda Franson

Testimonial

"*My Accidental Diet is a book full of inspiration; a delightful step by step guide on how to find your way back to health. Rhonda's story made me laugh and cry and it challenged me to start examining some of my own 'excuses' for not doing what I know serves my greater good. My Accidental Diet will take you on a journey full of wisdom, insight, vulnerability and practical tips that can easily be incorporated in to our day to day life. This book is a MUST read for anyone who finds themselves wondering how they can get on the fast track to feeling good again.*
Patti Fleury, BCR, CHN, Restoration Health (restoration-health.ca), author of Life After Crohn's: 5 Steps to Total Wellness.

"*Love, Love, Love this book. My Accidental Diet is the last book you will ever need to have on the issue of weight loss - a must read for anyone and everyone who has ever thought about or has ever been on a diet. Rhonda shares her story in such a way that you too can have the success she has had with weight loss. Prepare to be inspired. Prepare to be motivated.*"
Dianne Wyntjes

"*So inspiring and helpful to read Rhonda's book in the middle of my own health journey. She is proof that Life Change and Weight Loss are possible after 50! I can hardly wait for her cookbook. I follow her on Instagram too - she posts some delicious recipes. You go grrrl!*"
Liane McLaren

"As a personal trainer and group fitness instructor for the past 16 years, I often see women who have tried every diet in an attempt to lose weight. I'm delighted that Rhonda shows us in this book how to change our eating and fitness habits and achieve this without yo yo diets. I particularly love her recipe suggestions and food tips to replace the sugary deserts we all love!"

Rebecca Harrison. Best selling author, Personal Fitness instructor.

"As a health care professional I work daily with aging patients who suffer from poor health and limited mobility. I love that Rhonda made a decision to take control of her declining health through nutrition and exercise. It is possible. This book is full of inspiring stories not only for those wishing to lose weight but also for those people who want to improve the overall quality of their health. Proper diet and exercise are important components of health and are far too often overlooked.

As a friend of Rhonda's, it has been a wonderful journey watching her give birth to this book. She has been an encouragement to me personally. She walks her talk."

Shelley Neufeld, Nurse

Acknowledgements

Like most people, my life has been shaped and molded by the multitude of people I have met and the experiences I have had along the way. I am who I am because of these people and these experiences. So many people have touched my life in small ways and in big ways and for that I am forever grateful. There are several people, however, that I need to especially thank for their contribution to my life during the process of writing this book.

First and foremost, I need to acknowledge my husband Lyndon. I will never be able to thank you enough times for working diligently to keep our family afloat while I struggled to redefine myself. I know that you sacrificed a lot so that I could pursue my dream and for that I will always be grateful. I only hope that someday, some way I can repay you for all the love, sacrifice and support that you have given me and our family over the last several years.

To my son Conner: you have inspired and motivated me in ways you will never know. Thank you for pushing me to write you a story when you were just nine years old. Thank you for pushing me to run faster. Thank you for all your motivational *you can do it* speeches. Thank you for reminding me that the only limits are the ones we put on ourselves. You are an amazing human being. I am so proud of you and I am blessed to be your mom.

Speaking of moms, I need to say a special thank you to my stepmom. In my book I refer to her as my stepmom to differentiate between her and my birth mother. But, she has been 'Mom' to me since I was nine years old. She taught me many valuable life skills and for that I am grateful. She also gave me the best advice I received while writing this book. During a time when I was feeling like I just wanted to 'get the thing done', she told me that I needed to change my thoughts and reminded me that the reason I was writing the book was because I wanted to help a lot of people! Yes, Mom, you are right, I do want to help a lot of people! Thank you for the reminder – I needed that!

I also need to thank all my sisters and brothers who have encouraged me, shared experiences with me and never stopped believing that I would make my dream come true. You have all contributed in different ways and for that I feel blessed. I love you all so much. In particular I need to thank my sister Allona for being a huge inspiration to me on my fitness journey and to my brother David for sharing his own journey with me and for inspiring my final chapter.

To my friends: thank you! I especially need to thank Sabina Kramer. Without her, I don't know if I would be where I am today. She lovingly and generously shared so many life-changing tips with me during the miles and miles that we walked. I learned so much from you and you planted so many seeds of wellness in me that I will eternally be grateful for your knowledge, your enthusiasm, your support and your friendship. You are more than a friend, you are a teacher of wellness and I am blessed that I was one of your students.

To my friend Shelley Neufeld: thank you for being the best cheerleader a person could have! I mean seriously, how many people will run a marathon to help make someone else's dream come true? Thank you for running with me, for listening to me, for laughing with me and for talking me down when I was flipping out. Thank you for celebrating life with me. You are a good friend and I am so happy that we met.

To my life-long friend Shawna Stonehouse Lawson: we shared a lifetime of experiences when we were younger. Through those experiences you taught me determination and persistence. You also taught me how to make a 'sensational spinach salad'. Thank you for sharing your recipe and allowing me to add it to my book.

To my friend and holistic nutritionist Patti Fleury: you are such an inspiration. I was so happy that we reconnected on Facebook a few years ago and it has been a thrill and a privilege watching you grow your business and then go on to write and publish your own book. I think it is amazing that you healed your Crohn's disease and I lost my excess weight by changing many similar things in our diet and lifestyle. We may be onto something here! Thank you also for sharing your Almond Date Dark Cocoa Ball recipe with me and allowing me to print it in my book.

Early in my journey I read two books that greatly influenced me and taught me so much: *Wheat Belly* by William Davis MD and *Sexy Forever* by Suzanne Somers. These books changed my way of thinking and were the springboard for many changes that I made. I am so grateful to these two authors for sharing their knowledge and passion for food, health and wellness. My life is forever changed.

I have also been inspired by several accounts on Instagram. To name just a few: Angela Liddon @ohsheglows, Dr. Rachel Schwartzman ND @rachels_nd, Alyssa Rimmer @simplyquinoa. These people inspired me to try new recipes and opened doors to whole new ways of eating. Thank you for sharing your passion and inspiring the world with what you do. I am grateful I stumbled upon your accounts.

I have many people to thank who have been inspirational on my fitness journey. There are countless instructors, teachers, fellow students, business owners, friends and acquaintances that all helped me along the way. I especially need to thank my Bootcamp friends, everyone from the Abbotsford Running Room and all the amazing people from Haven Yoga and Wellness. These people are the best and I wouldn't be where I am without their guidance and support.

I also need to thank several people for reading my manuscript and giving me suggestions to make it better. Shelley Neufeld, my sister Dianne, my brother David and his life partner Liane McLaren all gave me valuable recommendations to make my book a better read. I need to give Liane an extra shout-out because of the edits that she suggested. She questioned me, called me out and asked for more. She made me think outside of my own brain and for that I am grateful.

My proofreader Lee Robinson deserves a huge thank you! I thought I had done a pretty good job of editing my book before turning it over to her; apparently not! Thank you for your patience with me, for your extra care and attention and for taking my words and adding the 'music'! I am truly grateful for all you did to take my book to the next level. You are a true professional and I thank you!

Some of the photographs in the book were taken by me, but many were not. I need to give credit to the following people for taking and sharing these photos with me:

Front cover: Bailey Marshall @breezy.bai. Thank you for answering my 911 call and for being available at a moment's notice. Thank you for your generosity, your talent, your extra effort and for being so fun to work with! You are awesome!

Front cover inspiration, photos on page 49 and 197, and author biography photo on page 225: Liane McLaren @liane_mclaren. Thank you for all the photos you took of me and for generously sharing your time and your talent to capture me in my happy places. You are the best!

Photo on page 22: Lyndon Fransoo. I died a little when I saw that picture of myself. I had no idea I was that big. But, I am happy I have the photo to remind me of how far I have come.

Acknowledgements

Marathon Finish Line photo, page 190: taken by MarathonFoto.

Body Composition Chart, page 26: The Competitive Edge.

The front cover was designed by Judith Mazari. I am so grateful to Judith for all the patience and support she showed me while designing the front cover. We went through several drafts before making the final selection. I am grateful for her creativity and expertise in bringing my foggy vision into clarity.

I would also like to thank Marilyn Wilson for her support in setting up and launching my book on social media.

Finally, I need to thank Julie Salisbury and Greg Salisbury from Influence Publishing. Thank you for your guidance, your patience and for answering my millions of questions. You brought my book from drab to fab and I am so grateful for all you did to help me out. I learned a lot in the process and I am so happy with the outcome. I could not have done this without your expertise and your never-ending support. Thank you from the bottom of my heart!

Contents

Introduction

Monday, January 5th, 2015

"As I come down the stairs, I can feel my heart beating and there is an uncomfortable anxiety flowing through my veins. It's not a bad thing. I know it is good because I am pushing myself out of my comfort zone. I have decided that this is the year that I will write my book and I am scared, to say the least. I am afraid of failure, I am afraid that no one will buy my book. I am afraid that I won't finish it. I am afraid it won't be good enough. I think that's the biggest fear....that it won't be good enough. But, as I write, I realize that is old language, old memories, and old stuff that I really need to let go of. I am good enough, my recipes are good enough, and my story is interesting enough to be told. In my heart I know that I have a story that needs to be shared. It happened to me for a reason: so that I can share it with other people. I see people suffering everywhere and I don't know how else to help other than by opening my heart and putting the words on paper that flow through me."

As I reread the paragraph above that I wrote on January 5, 2015, there are a few key phrases that stick out to me:

- "I am afraid of failure."
- "I am afraid it won't be good enough."
- "...so that I can share it with other people."
- "I see people suffering everywhere and I don't know how else to help other than by opening my heart and putting the words on paper that flow through me."

So, the time has come to set aside my fears and share my story to the best of my ability. In my book I will tell you how I lost 45 pounds, what changes I made, and how I made those changes a part of my everyday life. I need to clarify that I am not a nutrition specialist or a certified fitness instructor or a wellness coach. Because of my lack of certification I sometimes fear that my credibility will be questioned: *"Who is she to claim such things?"* But, the truth is that I am someone with a great deal of experience and along the way I have learned a lot. Over the course of my life I have been on several diets with limited, short-term success. I have lost and then regained weight many times. I have participated in many forms of exercise, again with limited fleeting success. Although I have always been interested in health and fitness I have certainly not always been a poster child for living a healthy lifestyle. I have abused my body time and time again. But, one day in the spring of 2013, my life was turned upside down and I was left sitting in a pool of confusion, anger, fear, resentment and so much self-doubt. My train had come off its track, and as I sat and watched the chaos around me, I felt a nudge that told me I had been on the wrong train!

So, after I cried and licked my wounds, I had no choice but to stand up and assess my situation.

What I saw was a very unhealthy person. Actually, what I saw when I looked around was a lot of unhealthy people. I knew I had to do something or my health would only continue to decline until I ended up in an early grave. I believe that our health is the most important thing we have and yet, when I looked in the mirror, my reflection told a different story.

I knew the time had come to regain my health, so I made a decision to start to take better care of myself. I knew that going on another diet was not the answer. I had already done that several times and I knew what the outcome would be. *No!* I needed to do something different: I needed to focus on health and well-being. So, I embarked on a journey of discovery and along the way I unearthed many new and exciting things about myself, about the body I reside in and about how food and fitness affect our well-being.

Among other things, I discovered that I like to cook and that I can actually put together some pretty decent, healthy and delicious meals. I discovered new foods that I had previously never heard of before. I discovered that food can be your most important friend in your life; it can be honest, true, nurturing and supportive in the most wonderful ways. I discovered a new meaning to the word "diet". No longer does it mean deprivation, hunger and sacrifice. The word "diet" now means **D**elicious, **I**nvigorating, **E**nergizing, and **T**antalizing!

I discovered new forms of exercise, found strength that I never knew I had and uncovered flexibility in my body that I didn't know existed. I discovered that when I take time to take care of myself that I have more energy and more time to better take care of my family and do so many other things.

Finally, and probably most importantly, I discovered how to eat in such a way that I felt nourished and completely fulfilled, without feeling deprived of the goodness and joy of food. In a nutshell, I discovered a whole new me; one that had been hiding behind excess weight, baggy clothes, insecurity, self-doubt, and loneliness.

By making a decision to take better care of myself and focusing on health and wellness, I was able to shed layers of excess fat, and in doing so I also discovered a whole new level of confidence and happiness. When I look in the mirror now, I like who I see. I don't think it matters if you have 20 pounds to lose, 40 pounds, 80 pounds or 180 pounds. The struggle is real for all of us who carry the burden of excess weight. We are all in a constant battle with food, we struggle with self-acceptance, and we feel trapped and out of control. Maybe we can't look at ourselves in the mirror because the reflection tells a story that we cannot believe. Regardless of your starting point, our bodies are all saying the same thing: "Too much is too much".

If you are at the point in your life where you want to embark on a journey to find a new you, then my hope is that by reading this book you will be inspired to make some positive changes to the way you eat and how you treat your body. I hope that you uncover that inner strength and beauty that makes you unique and special and that you use your unique set of life circumstances to guide you on your journey.

Take control of your health now so that you can live the best possible life, fulfilling all your hopes, dreams and desires. Our health really is the most important thing we have; we have to stop taking it for granted. We have to take control and make better decisions regarding our health and well-being.

I was asked to define what 'healthy' means to me. Over the course of my life 'healthy' has meant many different things. At one time I considered whole wheat bread and pasta to be 'healthy'. I considered 'fortified and enriched' boxed cereals to be 'healthy'. I thought the fact that I didn't drink soda pop meant that I was 'healthy'. The list goes on.

Being 'healthy' now means that I am taking care of my body, my mind, and my soul. It means being happy and joyful and being filled with gratitude for all the blessings in my life. It means being active and living out my dreams. It means embracing the day and trusting that my journey in life will continue to grow and evolve.

Introduction

A while back I had two words pop into my head: 'healthy body.' Right after that I thought: 'heal-thy body'! Then I understood that my job was to *heal **my** body*!

But, I can't stop there because I also need a healthy mind (heal thy mind). I also need a healthy soul (heal thy soul). I want a healthy family (heal thy family).

For me, 'healthy' is about healing.

My journey started many years ago and this is my story of how I finally lost the excess weight that was holding me back most of my life. Writing this book is much more than a deep desire to share what I learned. I feel it is my duty, my obligation to share my story. I believe that we all have stories and lessons that we have learned and that when we share those stories we help other people, and isn't that part of the human purpose?

I hope that by sharing my story that I will help someone, maybe a few people. I hope that my words will become a vehicle to guide you on your own personal journey towards health and wellness.

"It's not about going on another diet.
It's about discovering a whole new side of food and fitness.
And ultimately finding a whole new side of you."
Rhonda Fransoo

Chapter 1

I Wish You Knew How Beautiful You Are

I assume that because you are reading this book you are interested in losing weight. Maybe you have a hunch that losing a few pounds will help you improve the quality of your life and you want to know where to start and how to do it. Honestly, I hesitate to use the word **"diet"** in the title of my book because I don't want people to think that this is a diet book in the typical format. This is not a "how to lose weight" book. It is not a step-by-step program promising that if you do what I did, then you will successfully lose weight and keep it off.

The truth is that I can't tell you how to lose weight because I don't know you. I don't know your lifestyle, your likes, your dislikes, your strengths, your weaknesses. I don't know what you do for a living, if you are married or single, how many children you have, if you have any, where you live, what you do with your spare time, or who your friends are. So, how can I possibly tell you how to lose weight? The truth is I can't. I am sorry if you are disappointed. But, please don't put the book down and walk away. I have much to share.

My Accidental Diet is the story of how I lost 45 pounds. But, it is not about a diet that I went on, at least not a "diet" in the traditional sense.

Ironically, I did not start my journey with a goal of losing weight; I started with a need to improve my health and well-being and ended up losing 45 pounds, quite accidently!

But, before I get started on my story, I want to talk about you. I will start by telling you that you are an amazing and beautiful person! The fact that you exist is nothing short of a miracle. I think that most people don't even think about how amazing they are. Our bodies are a labyrinth of systems and intersections and byways and freeways all co-existing in the same unified body we call ourselves. Our bodies are complicated and intricate and fascinating beyond comprehension.

We walk around with these amazing pieces of biological machinery every day and give little thought to what makes them work; what makes them do all the things that we need them to do from breathing, thinking, walking, sleeping, laughing, reacting and lifting, to eating, digesting and eliminating.

Everything we do in our lives requires our bodies to do it! We don't physically exist without our bodies. Yet, how many of us actually sit in wonder and amazement at how beautiful and unique and truly awesome we really are? Not only are our bodies unique from each other, but so too are our dreams, our goals and our lifestyles.

If your purpose in reading this book is because you want to lose weight or improve your energy or your overall health then I want you to understand that your journey will be different from mine. You may not agree with some of what I say and that's the way it should be. For instance, I have chosen to eliminate about 80% of the wheat products from my diet. This works for me. If you don't agree with this, don't like the idea, or think I am crazy, that's okay, don't do it. Take the tidbits of information that speak to you, try them out, and then disregard the rest.

My hope is that you are inspired to walk down new roads on your way to a healthier lifestyle: that you discover new ways of thinking about food and exercise, and that you learn to trust yourself and learn to listen to what your body is telling you. My wish for you is that the positive changes that you make will last a lifetime and not just 21 days, 30 days or six weeks.

I hope you read this book with your heart and mind wide open, that you are inspired to ask questions, to look inside and to make changes based on your ability and lifestyle. I will tell you how I lost my weight, but, I can't tell you how to lose your weight because losing weight is not a *one plan fits all* process.

I think far too many people give their power away thinking that someone else has the answers. They follow complicated programs that will have them throw out every unhealthy thing in their kitchen, shop for a list of ingredients that they have no clue what to do with, count calories, count steps, fill in tedious "daily progress" charts, or follow complicated menu plans. Don't get me wrong, I think there is goodness in all these ideas and the intention is to help you. But, the problem is that they aren't designed for real life, they aren't designed for you and they aren't sustainable.

Eliminating unhealthy foods from your kitchen should be the goal, but eliminating without replacing them with alternative, delicious choices only leaves a gap that you will fill one way or another. We all like special treats and comfort food so we need to find new, healthy foods to replace some or all of our unhealthy favourites. You can't just toss things out and expect that to solve the problem; it doesn't. By no means am I suggesting that you go cold turkey and replace your favourite potato chips with kale chips; that would be an absurd suggestion and I wouldn't do that to you. Implementing progressive, small changes, one at a time, will set you up for success.

Shopping for new and healthy ingredients is a great idea too, but you have to know what to do with them. Just buying all the ingredients and letting them sit in your pantry or fridge doesn't solve the problem. You have to learn new ways to use these ingredients in your everyday meals. I added new healthy ingredients to my shopping list one at a time. This way I had time to learn how to incorporate them into my meal plans without overwhelming myself.

Counting calories and counting steps, in my opinion, should not be done. I get it, I have done both. The goal is to decrease your caloric intake while upping your activity. Obviously the goal is perfect, but, the tedious task of counting calories and steps is a waste of your precious time. Don't kid yourself into thinking this is the ticket to weight loss and fitness: it's not! Instead, eat real food (not processed, pre-packaged or fast food) and move your body and you will never have to count another calorie or step again. I have heard stories of people walking around their sofa during television commercial breaks so that they can get their goal steps in for the day – really?! Please don't do that. If you want to watch TV then sit down and enjoy your program. Better yet, record the program, go for a walk, then come back and watch your program at a later time when you can fast-forward through the commercials.

Filling in "daily progress" reports or food diaries is also a great idea because I do believe it is important to really become aware of how much water you are drinking, how many servings of fruits and vegetables you are consuming, how much bread you are eating, how many pieces of cake, how many ice cream cones and how many lattes you are enjoying in any given week. Awareness has power and it opens the door for change. However, I wonder how many people are 100%

honest when filling in those charts? I know I wasn't always honest; I cheated on the charts many times. I could never admit to eating a *"whole bag of chips"*, but I could admit to eating *"chips"*. The other problem with the charts is that I think far too many people spend too much time fussing over the charts and graphs and diaries. Life is busy. My thoughts are: spend that hour outside taking a nice long walk. You will feel great, much better than dealing with the fact that you never recorded that second helping you had at dinner, or that extra cupcake, glass of wine, or that peanut butter and jam sandwich which you accidently, on purpose forgot to record!

Finally, I want to talk about set diet plans. There are several of them: 30-day plans, 21-day quick-fix plans, 10 days to a new you plans, plans that promise you will lose 10 pounds in seven days! The list goes on: high protein, low carb, low fat, high fat, and no fat plans. They all sound so good and so promising; however, I have seen multiple times where people start these plans with the greatest intentions but then real life gets in the way and before too long the plan has derailed. I know from personal experience that sticking to someone else's menu plan and shopping list is not even remotely realistic. I have tried to follow weekly meal plans and I have failed every time. These plans don't take into account our individual likes and dislikes, they don't know our schedules, our budgets, our taste or our family lives. It is completely unrealistic to follow someone else's plan. You need to live within your own means and lifestyle and slowly adopt new, easy, healthier ways that work for you.

Another drawback of trying to follow a set menu plan is the fallout when you fall off the plan. We have all been there: Monday to Wednesday you follow the plan precisely, Thursday you go out for lunch and you have to order something off the menu which happens to be *"off the plan!"* Friday rolls around and you are exhausted and you order dinner in because you just can't deal with all the prep that goes into following a meal plan that was not designed for your lifestyle in the first place. By Saturday you give up because you have already blown your week. On top of that you start to feel bad about yourself for failing and then vow to **start fresh again on Monday morning**!

If you happen to be one of the few people who successfully make it through a regimented plan, then you obviously have a desire and a certain level of commitment to improve the quality of your health; for that you should be proud. However, the problem lays in the fact that during this time you haven't really learned how to integrate new healthy patterns into your routine in a way that suits you and your lifestyle. What you have done is shown perseverance and dedication to someone else's plan and long term that won't work for you. You can't follow someone else's plan successfully for a lifetime and still remain true to yourself. Of course I am assuming that you want the change to be something that lasts a lifetime and not just for a week, 10 days, 21 days or a month. There is no quick fix, no one-for-all plan, no guaranteed formula, and no magic pill. I believe that you, and only you, can design a plan that works for your life.

Of course, you need ideas and inspiration and a cheering section to help you along the way. In no way can I take credit for my weight loss on my own. I read books and I followed accounts on Instagram that promoted healthy eating and fitness and offered positive motivation. I tested new recipes, I took fitness training courses and I learned from people who were experts in their field. I was a hunter and a gatherer and I pieced together a new way of living that worked for me.

Many people have asked me how I lost my weight and when I start to tell them I usually get the look of *"oh please tell me something different; I don't want to hear that!"* Nobody really wants to hear: *"Well; I changed the way I ate and I started to exercise!"* No one wants to hear that because we are creatures of habit, we like comfort. We are afraid of change and it seems too overwhelming to change too many things. Plus, I think naturally we are all a bit lazy...come on... who doesn't prefer to be snuggled up on a couch watching a movie with a bowl of hot, buttered popcorn on a cold, winter night? Who wants to put on layers of clothes and head outside for a run when the air is so cold that you can see your breath and your teeth are chattering because you are frozen – who wants to do that!? Not too many people. The truth is you don't have to go to these extremes but you will have to make some decisions that at first will be really hard. But, each time you make a choice to step outside of your comfort zone and do something that pushes your boundaries, you will gain confidence and strength and you will be proving to yourself that you have what it takes to be successful, to reach your goal, whatever that might be.

To this day, there are times when I really, really don't want to go outside and run in the wind and the rain or the snow. There are times I am actually downright grumpy about the whole thing. I have to remind myself over and over that I will be fine once I start to run and that I will be so happy when my run is complete. I focus on the end result, and those happy thoughts pull me out the door and get me on my run. Never once have I ever regretted going for a run. On a couple of occasions I have actually got to my run and then changed my mind. No matter what I did, or how much I focused on the positive outcome of the run, I just couldn't do it, so I turned around and went home and tried again another day. I don't dwell on the fact that I missed my run. I give myself permission to listen to my body and be okay with what it is telling me. Some days, I just can't do it, and that is okay.

Yoyo dieting and binge exercising is a vicious cycle with no way out, at least not until you decide you want out. You have to take back the control and become the boss of your body, the CEO of YOU! You have to make a plan, learn new healthy recipes and find new and fun ways to move your body that challenge and invigorate it. You have to decide that you want off the roller coaster of weight loss and weight gain. Mostly, you have to learn to honour yourself and that beautiful, amazing body of yours.

There are many, many resources to help you on your journey. I hope that this book will become one of them. But, don't stop with this book; read lots of books, talk to people, go to lectures, watch healthy cooking shows, try different recipes. I will share some of my recipes and meal ideas that worked for me. These are not step-by-step plans that need to be followed day after day. Instead, I hope to inspire you to try new ways of pulling together healthy meals that fit your lifestyle. Nobody is asking for perfection, so forget about it, it doesn't exist. You are going to make mistakes. You are going to have a bad day, maybe a bad week. There will most likely be setbacks and you might have to start over again many times. That is part of the journey. That's how we learn. That's how we find out what works for us and what doesn't.

I am far from perfect in how I eat. I have weaknesses and I make unhealthy choices sometimes, and sometimes I love that I don't follow a set of rules and I can be rebellious and get away with it – at least for a while! But, when my rebellion turns into a habit – well, that's when things start to go sideways. I gain weight, lose energy and motivation, and start beating myself up for my stupid choices….no worries!! I have also learned not to stay on that destructive path. I have learned that I am only one choice away from getting back on my healthy journey and I know I can make one healthy positive choice. Then after that choice, I can make another and another and before I know it I am back on track, going forward, feeling good, feeling energetic and happy and proud of myself again.

My dream is that you discover new ways of doing things that work for you: that you start to move your body in ways that you never thought possible. I hope you discover that tiny, little voice inside your heart that nudges you down the path towards health, happiness and vitality. I want you to discover the joy of putting on your favourite jeans and realizing that they are too baggy. I want you to put on your shorts from last summer and experience the thrill of watching them fall to your ankles. I want you to pull out your little black dress and realize there is no way you can wear it to the upcoming event because it is way too big. I hope you experience the exhilaration of running up two flights of stairs and discovering that you can still talk when you get to the top. I want you to *experience the joy* of these moments because there is no way to explain it. These moments all happened to me and they filled me with 1000 times more happiness than any slice of seven-layer chocolate cake ever will!

I want this for you too; you deserve this. I know the challenges are real. I have been where you are. I have tried many diets in my lifetime and each and every one of them ended the same; I lost weight and then I gained it back!

Diets don't work. Again, I apologize for the title of the book, but I had to get your attention somehow!

Chapter 2

My Weight Loss Journey, but First, Some Background

I have been asked by many people how I lost my weight. There is not a simple answer to this question because the truth is that I did not set out to lose 45 pounds. My journey did not start out as a weight loss journey. I didn't wake up one morning and decide *"today's the day."* My goal was to improve my health, so there were many things that I did to bring about my weight loss. My journey was slow and unplanned and it happened over a period of several years as I discovered new ways of eating, exercising and taking better care of myself and my needs.

I can hear you say, *"YEARS! I don't have years; I need to lose weight now!"* I hear you; I have had special occasions that I wanted to lose weight for too. But, the truth is that it most likely took several years of repeating the same patterns and making the same choices to get you in the position you are in today. Like I discovered, those old patterns and ways of living can't be changed overnight. It is a process of discovering, learning and implementing new healthier ways. I will share the discoveries I made and the things I learned, but before I do, I want to start at the beginning so that you can get an understanding of my background and of the obstacles I faced and how a chain of events and decisions brought me to where I am today. I am a firm believer that everything happens for a reason so as I share my stories I want to be crystal clear that I hold nothing against anyone in my life past or present.

I love my story, where I came from and where I am going and I am grateful for the experiences and the support I have been shown along the way.

Growing Up

I was born in Red Deer, Alberta on March 29, 1962. At the time I had two older sisters and an older brother. When I was 5 years old my parents separated and my younger, three-year-old sister and I went to live with our mom in British Columbia. Actually, we didn't go to live with her; the truth is that she basically abducted us one day while our dad was away at work and we were at home with our three older siblings.

It is a long story, but for now I will talk about the four years that we lived with her. Those four years were a roller coaster ride of dysfunctional events: my mom had too many boyfriends, too many black eyes, drank too much booze, lied to us too much and left us alone way too many nights. We moved too much, went to too many schools and experienced too much loneliness. My life was full of fear and uncertainty.

During this four year period my mom had two more children: a daughter, Dorothy and a son, John. I was often left with the responsibility of caring for my three younger siblings. I remember having to take care of meals and bedtime on a regular basis as my mom and her boyfriend were often out late at night. My meals usually consisted of macaroni and cheese or soup and crackers. These meals were not very healthy for sure, but it's all I had to work with. I was seven to nine years old and we were poor. I did the best I could.

I made mistakes, like the time I placed my two-year-old sister in a bath of super-hot water. I can still picture her screaming and crying as her feet hit the scalding hot water. Clearly, I had not tested the water prior to plunking my little sister into it.

However, I did master testing the milk in the baby bottles so that it was just right...not too hot, and not too cold. My youngest brother got the benefit of my experience.

There were way too many responsibilities placed on my shoulders at far too young of an age. My mother was absent a lot in my younger years, but I know that she did the best she could at the time. I wish things could have been different for her. However, even in spite of all the chaos, I have a few fond memories of her.

One particular lunch time meal when I was in grade one, I had come home for lunch and my mom was home. She had made me cream of mushroom soup with crackers. I remember taking my bowl of soup into my bedroom. There was a table set up in the corner and there I could eat my soup in comfort and peace.

I remember finishing the bowl of soup and going to my mom and asking for more. She teased me a little about eating a whole can of soup myself, but I did. The soup was comforting, warm and nurturing which makes me ask: *"Did I have more soup because I was hungry or did I have more soup because I needed comfort and nurturing?"*

I think I know the answer to that question now, but, I didn't know back then. It was a rare occasion when I felt like my mom was taking care of me, and I wanted more!

It took me years to figure out that much of my overeating was because

I was looking for fulfillment, or comfort, or peace, or companionship. I turned to food to make me feel better. I believe this is a common problem. Food makes us feel better, at least temporarily.

The summer that I was nine and my sister was seven we went back to live with our father and new stepmom. My other younger half-brother and half-sister were given up for adoption and it would be another 25 years before I saw them again. Meeting them all those years later was a wonderful gift. I do see them from time to time and they are happy, loving people who were raised by loving parents who could be there for them since our mother could not.

Life with my dad and new stepmom seemed to be pretty normal. At least the daily chaos and upheaval came to an end. But, my weight slowly started to climb.

My stepmom put me on my first diet when I was about 11 years old. I was over 115 pounds and was at the point where I could no longer fit into children's clothing; I had to shop in the ladies department. It was an awkward experience!

I remember being so embarrassed that I had to be on a diet. I would sit in humiliation crunching away on iceberg lettuce salad and celery sticks while the rest of the family ate regular meals.

I remember weighing myself every day and I had made up a graph so that I could track my progress. It was a gruelling experience. I would be happy on the days that I had lost weight and depressed on the days I gained weight, and so the roller coaster ride began.

In the end, I did lose some weight. I got down to around 100 pounds and I do remember people complimenting me and that felt good. But, I hadn't really learned how to eat properly. I had learned to tolerate salads without dressing and celery sticks without cheese spread on top. That's about it! In the end, a girl cannot live on celery sticks and salad alone.

In high school I took Polynesian dance classes for fun and exercise. I also took physical education classes throughout my high school years. Back then, Phys. Ed. was optional. These activities kept my weight intact and I remember weighing 127 pounds in grade 12. I remember thinking that was a lot because I had friends who were much slimmer than I was. I also viewed my friends as being smarter, more popular and more talented than I was. I struggled with self-confidence and always felt like I wasn't good enough. High school was not a good time for me.

In addition, my stepmom and I did not always get along. I had come from a chaotic background where there were no rules, only survival. Trying to adjust to a new life of rules, chores and high expectations was not easy. I rebelled a lot and I know I failed to please her many, many times. She worked full-time, so again I was given the chore of making evening meals for the entire family. I made very basic foods: potatoes with every meal, a frozen or canned vegetable and then a meat of some sort, often pork chops in mushroom soup or meatloaf. Of course we always had the filler of bread and margarine with every meal. Back then we had limited ingredients, old homemade cookbooks with recipes from days gone by and no internet! I did the best I could, but my confidence suffered and mostly I felt not good enough.

The Single Life

Right after high school a girlfriend and I moved to Edmonton. It was a much bigger city about 100 miles away from our home. We had a lot of fun: we ate, we drank, we worked, and we partied.

During that time I decided that I needed to lose some weight again so I joined a weight loss company. Each morning I would take the bus to the weight loss coach's home for my weigh-in. It was time-consuming, expensive and the food choices were very limiting, but I was doing what I thought I had to do to lose the weight I had gained.

I recall one particular week when I hadn't lost any weight and she put me on the *"egg and grapefruit diet."* For three days all I could eat was eggs and grapefruit!

Can you imagine opening your lunch in front of all your coworkers in the lunch room and the smell of hardboiled eggs hits the room like a sulphur bomb? It was embarrassing to try to explain why I was only eating eggs and grapefruit!

How ridiculous!

Have you ever done anything like that?

The outcome of that diet was that I did lose some weight but by the following weekend I was done! I was like a ravenous bull.

I remember grabbing the can of whip cream from the fridge and spraying the whipped cream on crackers and stuffing my face like an out-of-control beast.

It makes me laugh to think of it now, and I can still see the whipped cream on my face and on my hands as I stuffed cracker after cracker into my mouth!

Apparently, eggs and grapefruit do not have all the nutrients that the body needs to live a sane and happy life! Obviously, whipped cream and crackers don't either!

What was I thinking?

Shortly after this experience I decided to try a more realistic approach to weight loss. I joined a different well-known weight loss company and started to count calories. I recorded everything (well, almost everything....I didn't record all the adult beverages I was consuming every weekend as my girlfriend and I were living it up as two single girls in the big city). The food was limited and not what I normally ate. There was most certainly merit in learning to eat more vegetables and controlling portion size. But, if at the end of the meal, or the calorie intake or the end of the day, you are still feeling hungry and you can't concentrate on anything else besides what and when you are going to be able to eat again, then I think the lesson is lost.

If you learn to eat food that fuels your body with all the necessary nutrients, then you shouldn't feel hungry all the time.

Our bodies need food, no question! But, the quality, variety and quantity need to be balanced and realistic in order for you to be successful. Eating a diet of eggs and grapefruit or any other ridiculously limiting "diet" is not realistic and will not set you up for success!

Unfortunately, that diet plan had the same results as the first and second diet I had tried. I did lose some weight but then I gained it back again.

My roller coaster ride of weight loss and weight gain continued for years. I gained weight when I worked for two years in a well-known restaurant. We ate, we drank, and we had a blast. I lost seven pounds the January I decided to stop drinking and eating late-night pizzas.

After that month I slowly gained the weight back. Then I lost weight when I moved to another province for a few months and decided to focus on exercise. I found a video tape that I liked and I exercised to it day after day after day. Then I joined a gym and attended aerobic classes on a regular basis. Staying active worked great at keeping my weight down and for a few years I was at a comfortable, healthy weight.

Then in 1989, my boyfriend at the time was killed in a motorcycle accident. The tragic accident hit a lot of people really hard. I was devastated and could hardly function for weeks. I couldn't eat or sleep and I lost a lot of weight. I remember being back at 127 pounds. I liked this weight but it was really hard to sustain. As soon as I started to recover from the shock of his death, I started to eat. As soon as I started to eat, I started to gain weight again. I had recognized a pattern: in order for me to sustain a healthy weight I either had to exercise like a crazy person, virtually quit eating or suffer a devastating loss.

Obviously, none of these options are healthy or sustainable.

Marriage and Motherhood

When I met my future husband in 1999, my weight was hovering around 138-142 pounds. I knew I could stand to lose a few pounds but I wasn't worried about it.

I had taken up running and I could run 10km so I felt like I was doing great and I was happy with where I was at. My husband and I had a whirlwind, romantic courtship and we were married in August 2001.

Our first couple of years of marriage were a time of huge adjustment for me. We moved a couple times during our first two years together. I had quit running because I was trying to get pregnant and I was commuting long distances for work. My eating habits changed. Suddenly we were eating dinners together every night. Previously as a single person if I felt like having popcorn for dinner, that's what I did. As a married woman, I felt like I couldn't do that anymore. I was moving less and eating more; slowly the weight started to creep up.

By the time I conceived in November 2002, I weighed 160 pounds. That number shocked me and I was sure the doctor's scale must be wrong!

I was worried about weight gain during my pregnancy because two of my sisters had each had pregnancies where they gained 60 pounds. That terrified me! If I gained 60 pounds I would be 220 pounds. I couldn't let that happen.

I got through my first trimester with a three pound loss. It was not intentional; I just had a hard time finding foods that were appealing to eat. The smells and textures of many foods affected me greatly. But, once I got past the first trimester, my appetite returned and I was able to resume eating regular meals. I did, however, make a point of eating lots of fruits and vegetables because I knew they were loaded with all kinds of nutrients that would benefit my baby. I was 40 years old and pregnant for the first time. You can bet I put nutrition on the top of my priority list, and I am so happy that I did. I delivered my beautiful, healthy, seven pound, nine ounce baby boy in August 2003, and I weighed 178lbs: only 18 pounds gained during my nine-month pregnancy.

Two weeks after delivering my son I was back into my jeans and this made me very, very proud. When I look back at my eating habits during my pregnancy I can now clearly see that my healthy food choices were a huge contributing factor to my minimum weight gain and the health of my baby.

As every new mom knows, life with a newborn is a whole different ball game. The game changes again when they are toddlers. It changes again when you go back to work. It changes again when the children start pre-school.

Life was about my son, my job, my husband, my home and somewhere in there, I got lost. Everybody else's needs came before mine, which left very little time to take care of myself.

I could feel my clothes getting tighter, so, I just went out and bought bigger clothes.

It wasn't long before my clothes were all too tight and my energy was low and I knew I had to do something if I was to keep up with my toddler, so off to a weight loss group I went again!

I re-joined a program I had tried years before. However, the program had been revamped and sounded more flexible and promising. I stuck with the program for about two months.

During this time I started to plan afternoon snacks because I had identified that I couldn't make it from lunch to dinner without something to eat. Because I was following a point system, I wanted to have the most volume of food for the least amount of points. I chose to take an apple and a pear because that was big volume for a snack and only two points. The problem was that two hours after eating these two pieces of fruit I was starving again! It made no sense, but what was I to do? I was hungry so I reached for more food, usually a piece of bread which was probably another one to two points; I don't remember. I do remember that I was constantly obsessing over food, counting points, feeling bad about myself if I was over my point allotment for the day, and mostly I was feeling hungry most of the time.

Yes, I did lose some weight but, really…who was I kidding?

I knew these plans didn't work for me and I knew it was unrealistic to try to live my life like this. So, I quit the plan and I started to gain the weight back.

My next stop to try and take back control of my eating was to head to a naturopathic doctor. I was getting desperate and knew that dieting was not the answer for me. I figured that a naturopathic doctor would be able to help me identify foods that I should and should not be eating. The first thing she did was put me on an elimination diet and gave me several supplements to take. I don't remember the details but I do remember living on a very restricted "diet", which did lead to weight loss but honestly, I knew I couldn't live with such restriction. So I quit seeing her, and returned to my old ways of eating.

Shortly after relinquishing my hope for a successful weight loss the Christmas season of 2008 was upon us. I made the deliberate decision that Christmas not to worry about what I ate or drank. I decided to enjoy the season: I hosted a gingerbread house building/cookie exchange party with my son's friends and their moms. There was no shortage of goodies and we had a great time.

A couple weeks later we hosted a more adult-orientated, open house party and in keeping with tradition there was again no shortage of appetizers, chocolate and specialty cocktails. New Year's Eve rolled around and again more delicious, delectable food and more cocktails. It was an overload but I didn't care. I was having a great time and for the first time in a long time it felt great to eat and drink whatever I wanted to without worrying. And finally, I wasn't hungry all the time.

However, after the tree was taken down and all the decorations were put away and all my clothes were feeling tighter and tighter I decided that perhaps I should weigh myself. Much to my horror I weighed in at 178 pounds!!

But, this time I didn't have a baby in my belly!

Something was wrong. I knew my health was suffering because I wasn't sleeping well, my blood pressure was high and I was irritable most of the time.

I did not feel good.

The stress of being a busy, working mom and wife often saw me eating and drinking way too much.

My weight had peaked and my energy had plummeted.

I felt caught in a vicious cycle.

If I ate to satisfy my appetite, I gained weight. If I ate less, then I was hungry all the time. I knew something was wrong and I needed to make some changes.

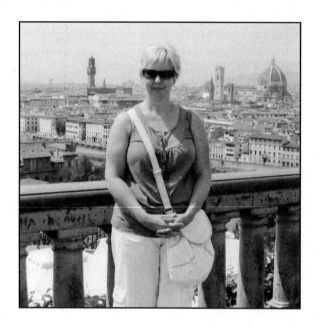

Summer 2009 while on vacation in Italy

My Journey Begins

My journey to improve my health and start to feel better began by identifying one thing: I got hungry at lunch time! How silly does this sound? You see, I was in the habit of not planning for lunch in the morning before I headed off to work. I worked as a sales representative and spent most of my day travelling from customer to customer. I rarely took scheduled lunch breaks because each day my route and appointments were different. I would start my day with a breakfast, usually consisting of a bowl of cereal and a piece of toast, not because I was hungry, but because I knew I needed to eat something for breakfast, I had heard over and over again that breakfast was the most important meal of the day....so, I ate breakfast and felt full and the thought that I would need more food by lunch did not enter my brain. But, sure enough, each and every day I would be starving by about 10:30 – 11:00.

This was my invitation to stop for a coffee and muffin and continue on my way. About an hour or so later I would be famished and need to stop for food again. I usually hit a drive-thru or grocery store to pick up some sort of sandwich or burger, which would usually satisfy me for a while. However, like clockwork, a couple hours later I would be hit with that same old feeling of *"I need something to eat and I need it now!"* The hunger pangs sent me once again in hunt of a quick fix usually consisting of another coffee and a donut or a chocolate bar. By the time I got home, I was hungry again and I usually snacked on crackers while making dinner. It was a constant roller coaster ride of being hungry, then full, then famished, then satisfied, then starving.

My day was consumed with food. I was clearly eating lots of food, but why was I so hungry all the time?

It finally occurred to me that indeed I did get hungry every lunch time and I always needed to stop for a snack in the afternoon. I decided it would probably be a good decision to start to pack a lunch that incorporated more vegetables and fruit. So, I purchased a wide-mouth thermos that I could put soups and stew in. The thermos would keep them hot and I knew if I added extra veggies to the soups and stews then that would probably be a good idea.

At first my soups were nothing more than a can of store bought soup to which I added lots of extra veggies and sometimes leftover chunks of chicken or beef. In my lunch I also packed a piece of fruit. This plan really worked. I found the warm soup/stew to be very satisfying and I felt so much better eating this than eating a sandwich. No longer did the mid-afternoon cravings take over my body and my better judgement. The trips through the drive thru almost came to an end.

This was successful.

The proof came when I found myself rushing out the door in the morning without packing my lunch and I ended up eating a burger or processed sandwich for lunch, and like clockwork the cravings would start all over again. I would be back repeating old patterns.

It took a few weeks of trial and error to figure out that being prepared with a nourishing lunch completely changed how I felt.

Changing just one bad habit started my weight loss journey:
I started to take my lunch to work.

Identifying the next flaw in my daily eating ritual came by accident. As previously mentioned, my breakfast of choice was usually a bowl of cereal and a piece of toast. Occasionally, I would have a bowl of oatmeal. It took some time for me to discover that on the days that I ate oatmeal I didn't have the mid-morning feeling of starvation and deprivation that I previously had experienced when I ate only cereal and toast. Clearly, eating cereal and toast didn't sustain me, so I made the decision to eat oatmeal more often. Just by changing these two things I lost about five pounds.

Those five pounds made a difference in the way my clothes fit which naturally made me very happy. Of course the trick was to make these changes a way of life. I discovered that if I stuck to eating oatmeal and took a healthy lunch and snack with me 80 – 90% of the time, I could sustain my weight loss. If I got lazy or I forgot or I was too rushed to plan, then I would feel my pants getting tighter and I would start to feel those hunger pangs starting all over again.

I had learned a few new things and I was starting to see some results. It was about this time that I started running again. I knew from past experience that exercising always worked wonders for me. However, I had neither the time nor the drive to exercise to the extent that I had in the past. But I did what I could, I laced up my shoes and went for a walk/run, sometimes only a few blocks, but the effort resulted in a further loss of a couple more pounds.

Over the next couple years my weight fluctuated between 168-172 pounds. Although I was far from my ideal weight, my clothes were fitting better and I had made a couple of positive changes.

However, in March 2012, I came face to face with the fact that although my efforts had resulted in some positive changes, I was still far from where I needed to be. Our local rec centre was hosting a mini trade show for local health and wellness companies. One of the booths I stopped at was offering free body composition analysis. I thought *"why not"* and stepped on the scale. The results shocked and troubled me. Yes, I knew I was overweight but being told I was "'stage 2 obese'" was a real slap in the face. However, the biggest shock was that my metabolic age read as 73.0 years old! I was only 49!

I didn't exactly know what that meant, but I was humiliated and knew that my health was clearly in jeopardy.

Name	Rhonda Fransoo	*Age/Gender*	49 Female
		Height	5-5.0 ft-in

Results

Weight	167.6 lb
Body Mass Index (BMI)	27.9
Body Fat %	42.6 %
Body Fat Mass	71.4 lb
Body Fat Range	Obese
Fat Free Mass	96.2 lb
Visceral Fat Rating	9
Body Water %	40.4 %
Body Water Mass	67.6 lb
Muscle Mass	91.2 lb
Bone Mass	4.8 lb
Basal Metabolic Rate	1351 kcal
Metabolic Age	73.0 yrs
Daily Calorie Intake	2107 kcal
Physique Rating	2-Obese

Body Composition Chart - March 2012

More Changes Coming.........

Sometimes we make changes in our lives and sometimes life makes changes for us. The latter happen to me in March 2013.

We were just finishing renovations on our house that we had bought three years earlier. My son was doing great in school, my husband had just completed an exceptional year at his work and I was working for my dream company. All was good, or at least on the surface it was good. The truth was that I was struggling with my job as a sales rep. No matter what I did, I could not increase sales; companies were closing, downsizing and reinventing themselves. I struggled with how to work my territory and I knew things were not good. I was stressed and although I was doing my best to take care of myself, I was failing at that too. Then one day, out of the blue, my contract was suddenly and abruptly terminated and I found myself unemployed for the first time since I was 17 years old!

To say I was devastated is an understatement. It was one of the most difficult times of my life. I knew I had been working my territory to the best of my ability; I was well respected and I knew my customers valued my service. I could not wrap my head around the fact that the company was telling me that I had no plan, that what I was doing was not good enough! It made no sense that they were letting me go! However, within the first few days of my termination I had a couple of events take place that reassured me that it all happened for a reason and that I would be okay.

The first thing that happened was that one morning as I sat down to eat my breakfast I had an unusual awareness come over me; I felt like I was tasting my food for the first time. It was a very strange sensation of being fully present in the moment. The house was silent, the phone was silent. There was nothing for me to do, nowhere for me to go. It was just me and my breakfast sitting face to face. I wondered how long I had been gobbling down my food without any awareness of the taste or texture of what I was consuming I wondered how long had it been since I last **tasted** my food? I had no idea .

The next incident happened a few days later. I was in the grocery store midday picking up a few things and I found myself leisurely meandering though the aisles. I chatted with a couple of people and once again felt very present in the experience: I was so much more aware of where I was and what I was doing. I had shopped during the day before but I was always in a rush to get to the next appointment or make the next phone call. I had never had a grocery shopping experience quite like that one. The sense of calm, the realization that I had nowhere to go, no one waiting for me to return a phone call, no problems to solve, no expectations from anyone. I was free and at peace to do my grocery shopping and to really be present in the experience. And although the tears were still flowing and the sadness was surrounding my being, I found hope and peace in these two amazing experiences and I knew I would be okay and that I was in the right spot in my life.

I knew I had lost my job for a reason.

Losing my job was a horrible experience, one I wouldn't wish on my worst enemy. However, I do now see in hindsight that it was one of the best things that ever happened to me. My world was shaken and when I finally caught my breath from the shake-up what I saw was truly life changing. Everywhere I went I saw people who were overweight, who looked unhealthy and who struggled with simple everyday tasks like climbing a few stairs. What I observed frightened and saddened me at the same time.

I knew I needed to do something or I was going to head further down the road I was already on: the road that lead to continued declining health and additional weight gains! It was time to pay attention; it was time to take care of myself. I had too many dreams yet to fulfill, too many things that I wanted to do and experience. I longed to be one of those people who were living active, fulfilling, inspiring lives. I wanted to feel better, look better and enjoy more that life has to offer. I had spent my life taking care of other people; it was time to take care of myself and to reclaim my health and well-being.

I believe most of us spend a great deal of our lives on automatic pilot, so much so that we become numb to our own feelings and actions. We just keep doing the same things over and over until one day life shakes our world and the automatic pilot button is shut off. When this happens we have no choice but to wake up and pay attention. We have no choice but to take control of our lives and steer our vessel in a new direction.

Losing control of my life was scary and it was hard and it hurt!

Taking back control was a day-by-day journey. I started off slow, making positive decisions and changes bit by bit. With each small successful step, my confidence grew, and then I started to feel better. My energy and zest for life started to return and I was finally able to start doing some of the things I had longed to do for years. A new 'me' was emerging and what I saw, I liked. So, I continued to learn and grow. Eventually, I reached a point where people started to notice and comment on my progress. They wanted to know what I did to lose my weight.

The idea came to me that I would like to share my weight loss story as a way of giving back and hopefully inspire other people to take control of their own health and well-being. And so this book was conceived.

Chapter 3

One Decision at a Time

Becoming aware of how unhealthy I had become was a gift to me. Being truly aware of the problem opened the door to finding solutions. I knew I was not prepared to go on a diet because I knew diets didn't work for me and frankly I didn't want to go on another diet. I didn't want to feel deprived and hungry.

What I wanted was to feel good, feel alive, and feel energetic. I wanted to live a long, active, healthy lifestyle. I wanted to make changes that I could sustain for the rest of my life.

I knew that many of the health issues I was facing (being overweight, high blood pressure, poor sleep patterns, and stress) were related to the food I was eating and the lifestyle choices I was making. I believe this to be true for many people who are facing health issues. I believe that food should be our medicine; instead it is becoming our source of toxicity and disease. We are burdening our bodies with unhealthy excess that they are struggling to deal with. I certainly knew this was the case for me.

I wanted something different. I wanted to be healthy and feel good, so that became my main focus. I started to ask myself, *"What would a healthy person do?"* This question became the springboard for a series of answers. The first answer I came up with was, *"Make one healthy choice decision at a time."* So, that is how I started the next part of my journey.

I remember one particular summer afternoon, a girlfriend and I had taken our boys to a nearby lake for the afternoon. The boys wanted to get some ice cream so we walked over to the ice cream stand and we ordered cones for our boys. My girlfriend also ordered and then asked me what I wanted. At that single moment I made a choice not to have an ice cream cone. I simply said, *"No thanks, I am going to pass today!"* She looked at me with a combination of bewilderment and pride and simply said, *"Good for you."* It is hard to describe how I felt at that moment. It was a moment of victory, a moment of triumph. I had said *no* to ice cream and I felt powerful. I hadn't said *no* to ice cream for the rest of my life, I hadn't said *no* to ice cream because I was on a diet! I simply said, *"No thanks, I am going to pass today"*. It was a small victory that lit a spark within me. It was a small building block to add to my new foundation.

I had a similar experience on another occasion early on in my journey when I had gone out for lunch at one of our local restaurants that served, in my opinion, the best hamburger and fries. In my past life I always ordered the same thing. I loved their burger and fries (and sometimes I also had a piece of seven-layer chocolate cake for dessert). But, on this particular day, I made the decision to order a salad instead of the fries! **Yes!** I felt triumphant.

I didn't order the salad because I was trying to cut calories. I hadn't ordered the salad because I was on a diet. I ordered the salad because it was a healthier choice than fries. I also ordered the salad because I was consciously choosing to break the unhealthy habit of ordering fries. Remember, my goal was to get healthy so I chose salad because it was a healthier choice. I still ate the burger and it was good, but the salad was good too. I hadn't made a choice to say goodbye to fries forever. I had made a choice to eat a healthy salad that day, at that moment.

This was another small victory that had a huge impact. I felt proud of my decision and my body felt good too. I have eaten fries since then, but honestly, when I do, I mostly wish I had ordered a salad. A salad always makes me feel better in the long run and feeling good and feeling strong and feeling healthy is my goal.

Another habit that I decided to change was the habit of *"having a little bit more"* at meal time. In my heaviest times I noticed that, at dinner time especially, I had the habit of going back for a second helping of food or *"just a little bit more."* I did this most of the time. Once I recognized my unhealthy pattern, I made a decision not to do this anymore. I told myself that if I thought I needed more food, then I had to fill my plate fuller on the first round, so that is what I did. However, once I saw how much food I was eating it became a great visual that it was too much. Somehow two smaller plates of food were acceptable but one large portion was not, so I cut down my portion size and stopped having second helpings. This was one more successful, positive step forward on my weight loss journey.

The other thing that I discovered after implementing the *"one serving only policy"* was that the *"20-minute rule"* is real, meaning that it takes 20 minutes for your brain to get the message from your stomach that you are full. By not loading up on a second helping of food, more often than not I found that I didn't need or want a second helping of food. By not overloading my body I had given it time to absorb the food and, consequently, my brain received the message that I was full. It made me wonder how long I had been overeating because I never gave my body the time to process the fact that I had eaten plenty and did not need any more food. Slowing down and backing away from the table was very important in my weight loss journey.

Remember what I said earlier, I didn't make all these changes at once. I changed things slowly. I just kept asking myself what a healthy choice might be, and I usually made that choice. Not only did I make choices about what and how much to eat. I also had to make choices about exercise. I had a friend who liked to walk after dinner. She often asked me if I wanted to walk with her. My first reaction was most often, *"No, I am too tired."* But, then I thought about it a bit more and knew that I would probably feel better if I walked, so off we went.

Those walks reminded me how great it felt to move my body and became the spring board for my future fitness endeavours. Over the course of the last few years I have had many times when I didn't want to walk or run or exercise, but I got into the healthy habit of asking myself:

"Did I want to feel good because I had exercised?"
Or
"Did I want to feel bad because I hadn't?"

The answer was clear: I wanted to feel good! So, off I went for a walk, or a run, or to exercise class. And you know what? Not once did I ever regret my decision! Not once! And more so, I always felt better after getting some exercise. It was good for my body and my mind.

As I made changes, my grocery shopping experience changed too. I would make a point of thinking about what healthy people would have in their shopping carts. As a result, I started to add more fruits and vegetables into my cart. I also made the decision to stay away from the aisle of chips, cookies, chocolate, pastries and pre-packaged, quick meals. I knew that healthy people would load their cart with good quality, nourishing food, not crap food. So, I did what they did.

It became a bit of a game for me. I loved it when I went through the till and the cashier would ask me what I was making with a particular item I was buying. I wanted to look the part of a healthy person, cook like a healthy person and use ingredients that healthy people use.

I wanted the healthiest cart in the store!

I know this probably sounds silly but it was a little motivational game I played with myself and it worked. I don't know if my cart was the healthiest cart in the store, but, I do know that this little game helped me make better and better choices as I continued on my journey. Ask yourself: "What is in your grocery cart?" "What can you add to make it healthier?" "What can you put back on the shelf and say 'no' to?"

I continued to make positive choices one decision at a time. I plugged away day by day. I tried new things, a lot of new things. I took time to read and to learn. I made new conscious choices and slowly, very slowly, I started to see changes in the way my clothes fit. I started to have more energy; I started to sleep better at night.

Then an amazing thing happened; people started to notice the changes in me. I will never forget the day I heard someone say to me, *"You are so little!!"*.......say what? *"Me? Little? What?!! You got the wrong person!"* It was as if they were talking to someone else, and I guess in reality I had become someone else. I had shed layers of fat, I had toned my body. I felt great and it must have shown! As I write these words I can't help but get emotional! It fills me with so much happiness.

I had finally learned new ways. I had finally broken the barrier; I had finally got off the vicious roller coaster ride of dieting. I finally had gained control and knowledge, and as you know: knowledge is power.

I wrote this book to share my story. I want this for you too. I want you to experience the thrill of victory, the pride of self-control and the joy of discovering a new happier healthier version of yourself.

The First Step in Your Journey

I know that starting a weight loss program, a fitness program, or a healthy lifestyle program can be overwhelming. There is so much information out there. Some of it is conflicting, it is confusing and I know from personal experience that sometimes the job seems too big, too complicated, and too difficult to start. But, if you want to change the quality of your life then start you must. Pick one single change that you can make, or take a single idea that you can implement and then do that one thing.

It really is that simple.

You can start your new healthy journey right now. You can put down this book and go for a walk right now! You don't have to commit to a 5 km walk or a lengthy program. Just go and walk for a block or two. This is a single positive choice that you can make that gets you out the door and on the road to wellness; it starts the momentum.

You could also stop reading right now and enjoy a glass of water. Drinking water is so good for you. Most people don't drink enough water and many people eat because they think they are 'hungry' when in fact their bodies are actually 'thirsty'. Do your body a wonderful favour and give it lots of water.

When I know I am not getting enough water I make a point of filling up my eight glasses of water in the morning. I flavour each glass with a different item, including blueberries, cucumbers, mint, strawberries, lemon, limes, or any other flavouring that I have available. I love my fancy water glasses, and I always drink all eight glasses when I do this little trick. It works for me.

Next time you go out for lunch order a salad instead of fries, or pass on the dessert.

Break the habit of having second servings at the dinner table.

Next time you crave a bag of chips, reach for an apple instead. It doesn't mean that you can't have chips again; it means right now, today, you choose an apple.

Make a point of adding one new healthy ingredient into your shopping cart each week. Maybe try a new vegetable that you have never had before. Check out the "health food" aisle and buy something new. Buy organic meat or poultry. Filling your cart with healthy foods will make you feel good. Preparing and eating those healthy foods will make you feel even better.

Start to think like a healthy person and then make your choices accordingly. There are so many choices to be made, so don't overwhelm yourself, just make them one at a time. Each positive, healthy choice you make will fill you with pride and a sense of triumph which will build your confidence and give you that "I got this" feeling. Each baby step takes you closer to the finish line and crossing the finish line will be one of the happiest moments of your life. Take a moment to breathe in what I am saying:

"Starting a wellness or weight loss program doesn't have to be all-consuming and complicated. It is just one healthy decision at a time."

Each healthy decision that you make is a building block in the foundation of your new lifestyle. Each successful baby step adds strength to your purpose, just keep making those positive decisions again and again, soon you will notice a difference in how you feel.

Then you will notice a difference in how you look.

Then other people will notice.

It doesn't happen overnight. It happens slowly. But, consider this: if for one year you made one healthy choice each day, at the end of the year that would be 365 healthy choices! Your body would absolutely feel the difference. So, don't wait until tomorrow to get started, do it now, do it today. Make one decision, but remember to be patient and be kind to yourself; after all, you are trying to undo a lifetime of habits and patterns that have not served you well. You are moving from unhealthy to healthy and it is a step-by-step process.

In closing this chapter, I think the single biggest piece of advice I can give you as you start your journey is to:

"Make one positive healthy choice decision at a time!"

That's what I did, and it worked for me.

Chapter 4

Discovering That Food Is Fuel

Controlling portion size, occasionally saying no to tasty treats, choosing a salad instead of fries and starting to walk/run again were all good healthy choices I made early in my journey. Each healthy choice that I made added to the momentum of my journey and kept me on track. The more success I had, the more I wanted. However, these were just a few simple steps that I took in the beginning of my journey. As I continued to ask myself, *"What would a healthy person do/eat?"* I found myself starting to think more and more about my food choices.

One of the things that I became aware of was that some days I would experience crazy hunger pains, shakiness and abdominal cramping, and other days I wouldn't. I honestly wondered if I was pre-diabetic or had some other eating or digestion disorder. A typical day would look like this:

8:00 am	Breakfast:	Cereal with milk and toast or oatmeal
10:30 am	Snack:	Muffin and coffee
12:00 pm	Lunch:	Sandwich, or burger and fries, or soup
3:00 pm	Snack:	Apple, pear, cookies or donut
5:00 pm	Pre-dinner:	Piece of bread or crackers & cheese

| 6:00 pm | Dinner: | Meat, potatoes, pasta or rice and vegetables |
| 8-9:00 pm | Snacking: | Chips, popcorn, or more crackers & cheese |

By the time I started to really take notice of what I was eating and how it was affecting me, I had already started to eat oatmeal occasionally for breakfast and I had started to take a thermos of soup or stew for lunch. It was on these days that I noticed that I didn't experience the *"I'm starving"* shaky sensation that overtook my body and my senses and often sent me to the nearest drive thru or convenience store. I realized that oatmeal actually satisfied me until almost lunch time and when I did get hungry I wasn't *"starving to death,"* I was simply hungry. This was fascinating to me and I started to wonder why this was happening.

Getting Some Answers

I have a strong belief that when we start to wonder about something and we ask questions about a particular subject, we will get the answers if we pay attention and listen. You know the old saying: *"When the student is ready, the teacher will come."* Sure enough, life delivered the answer to my question. One day during a long walk with a friend, she started to tell me about a book she was reading called *The Wheat Belly,* by William Davis, MD. On another walk she shared with me information she was reading in a book called *Sexy Forever,* by Suzanne Sommers. I decided to listen to my friend and I went out and bought these two books.

I gobbled up the information and then I read more books. I learned about macronutrients, micronutrients, protein, simple carbohydrates, complex carbohydrates, essential fats, and unhealthy fats. I learned that our bodies need a complex combination of all these things (except the unhealthy fat) in order to function properly.

I learned that because of the way our food is often grown, modified, processed, and packaged that many of the vital nutrients that our bodies need have been stripped away leaving much of our food with calories but very little else.

I read how genetically modified food is seldom recognizable in our bodies and how unrecognizable foods get stored because our body doesn't know what to do with these *"foods"*; it can't break them down, process them or benefit from them so the body just stores them.

It is scary to think what we put in and on our bodies day after day without really thinking about it!

The aha moment came for me when I finally discovered and came to understand the thing called *"blood sugar levels."* I always knew that sugar was bad for me and I felt blessed that I was born with a *"salt-tooth"* instead of a *"sweet-tooth."* I would sooner have a bag of chips than a chocolate bar any day. Not that I didn't eat chocolate bars, I did. But, I preferred salty crunchy snacks over sweets. I thought I was doing well because I didn't consume a lot of sugary products, including pop: I rarely drink the stuff. However, what I didn't know was how carbohydrates react in our bodies.

I learned that when we ingest carbohydrates they turn into glucose (sugar) in our blood stream. When this happens, our brain releases insulin (insulin is the fat storage hormone). The insulin rushes to the sugar and converts it into fat and stores it in our cells for use at a later time. When we consume more carbohydrates than we are actively burning off, our bodies become storehouses for the excess carbohydrates (which converts to fat).

It really is a scary thing.

However, the good news is that not all carbohydrates are created equally. There are simple carbohydrates and complex carbohydrates.

In a nut shell, the simple carbohydrates (sugar, bread, muffins, pasta, cereal, pizza crust, bagels, cookies, and flour) enter our blood stream quickly and insulin is released rapidly. Once the sugar has been stored as fat, our body sends a message to our brain that our blood sugar levels are low and that more sugar is required: in other words *"that it's hungry!"* This explained why after eating cereal and toast in the morning I would be starving by about 10:00 am. The process of converting carbohydrates to fat takes approximately 90 minutes. This was amazing and valuable information for me.

Complex carbohydrates (whole grains like oatmeal, brown rice, quinoa, beans, peas, and lentils and most fruits and vegetables) on the other hand, take time to break down in the body and therefore do not enter the blood stream so quickly. This means that only small amounts of insulin are being released and therefore very little fat storage is occurring. This was truly fascinating to me.

Learning to eat in such a way that I could control my blood sugar level was a life changing discovery.

Armed with this new information I started to look at the food choices I was making and realized that even though I was not consuming large amounts of sugar and fats, I was consuming large amounts of simple carbohydrates in the form of cereal, bread, muffins, crackers and pasta. It seemed that the simple carbohydrates were messing around with my blood sugar levels and sending false messages to my brain that I was *"starving."* Furthermore, the excess sugar (from all the simple carbohydrates) was being stored as fat on my body. I then started to wonder if the cramping and bloating was also tied to the food choices I was making.

When I examined the list of foods that I was eating I concluded that I was eating too much of some things (simple carbohydrates) and too little of other things (complex carbohydrates, protein, and healthy fat). In essence my body was *"starving,"* but it wasn't more food that it needed, or at least not more of the food I was giving it. My body was getting plenty of food, but it was lacking the balanced combination of nutrients that my body was starving for, so my body used what little it could, stored what it couldn't and begged for more. What my body was actually begging for was proper nutrients: less simple carbohydrates, more complex carbohydrates, more protein and some healthy fat. It needed real, whole food; food that it could actually process, absorb and benefit from. It needed food that was fuel, not just filler!

It became clear to me that I needed to make some changes and so the first major decision that I made was to eliminate as many wheat products as I could from my diet! This included all my favourite traditional standby items like cereal, muffins, bread, pizza, cake, pasta and crackers. For me this was life-changing! (I know that right about now I am going to lose a few people but remember what I said at the beginning: you won't agree with everything I say and that's a good thing. Take what speaks to you and disregard the rest. This is your journey; I am just sharing my story and what worked for me.)

Eliminating wheat products may seem like a drastic move and I would agree that few of us would be happy and be able to sustain a diet that didn't include pancakes, pizza, pasta and cake! I mean really, who could do that? Eliminating these favourite food items was not the answer; however, replacing some of the ingredients in these items was the answer. I went to work to find new ways to make these favourite items by replacing most of the processed flour and refined sugar (simple carbohydrates) with ingredients that our bodies can actually benefit from (complex carbohydrates, protein and healthy fat).

It was a 'one-recipe-at-a-time' process. Initially I had a friend tell me about a chocolate cake she made that used quinoa instead of flour, then I heard about cauliflower pizza crusts, then I started to make homemade soups using squash and all kinds of other vegetables. I found creative ways to introduce a lot more complex carbohydrates into my diet. I especially added more vegetables, lots more vegetables: lots of colour. I had seen a hashtag on Instagram called *#eattherainbow*. I liked that. It resonated with me. Prior to this my meals were often beige and brown. Those colours lack vibrancy and vitality. Nature designed food in an array of glorious colours not only because they contain different vital nutrients, but also to tantalize us and invite us to enjoy their goodness. Each glorious colour offers the body something essential. Everything you need is found in the colours of the rainbow, so, stop chasing the rainbow and start eating it.

I also added more lean protein and healthy fats to my meals. One recipe led to another and before I knew it I was rarely eating any wheat products. I found that my crazy *"starving"* episodes were few and far between, my cramping and bloating had all but disappeared and the most exciting thing was that I started to lose weight.

I had started the process of fuelling my body in such a way that it was finally getting a balanced amount of the macronutrients and micronutrients that it needed and the reward was that my body was happier, healthier and slimmer. Not only did I start to lose weight but I started to sleep better, I had more energy and my blood pressure slowly started to decrease. Most importantly, I felt content and realized that sometimes I went for two, three, sometimes four hours without thinking about food! This was a miracle indeed! I thought: *"If the cells of my body could sing, I am sure they would have been singing **Hallelujah**"*. At the very least I knew they were whispering: *"Thank you – now we have something to work with."*

On my journey I changed many things about my eating habits, mostly, I changed my thoughts: I changed how I thought about food. I started to think of it in terms of how it would fuel my body. What was the purpose of the food I was eating? How would my body benefit?

I learned that a breakfast of oatmeal or scrambled eggs and vegetables fuelled me for hours and saved me from countless unhealthy drive-thru muffins and donuts.

I learned that a simple salad for lunch was not enough and would leave me hungry, but, that if I added some protein like some chicken chunks or egg, as well as some healthy fat like avocado or nuts, then I would feel satisfied for several hours.

I learned that two pieces of fruit for an afternoon snack would fill me up, but that I would be starving again less than two hours later. I learned that an apple and a few almonds were not as filling, but reacted in my blood stream beautifully and provided me with constant flowing energy for the remainder of the afternoon.

I learned how to make yummy and delicious chocolate and pina colada shakes that are chock-full of nutritious ingredients that my body gobbles up in delight.

I learned that depriving my body of the essential nutrients was equivalent to starving myself while carrying around an excess 40 pounds. Essentially I learned the difference between filling my stomach and fuelling my body. The latter became my goal.

I want to say again that I never went on a "diet." I also never felt deprived and the shaking feeling that I was about to starve to death all but disappeared. I figured out that my body was starving for nutrients and when I finally started to feed it the nutrients that it desperately needed, it rewarded me in ways I could only have dreamt of.

In short, I learned that our bodies are amazing, efficient machines, but most of us are really poor mechanics. We need to learn how our bodies work and then we need to take time to fuel it with the proper combinations and types of food. Most people treat their cars better than they treat their bodies; this needs to stop!

Start Your Engine!

Learning to fuel your body with life giving nutrients will change your life and may even save your life. On my food posts on my Instagram account I often use the hashtags *#foodisfuel, #foodismedicine and #foodislove*. I believe all this and more about food. I have learned a lot and have developed a whole new appreciation for the wonders of food. The sooner you start to view food in a new light, the sooner you will be able to make life-enriching food choices.

I share my story because I know that I am not alone here. When I look around at people I wonder how many people are actually starving themselves of vital nutrients. How many people go on weight loss plans and do great for a few days or maybe even a few weeks and then one day the old, ugly cravings creep in and they snack on a piece of cake, or maybe a cookie or 12. Maybe they rip open a bag of chips and shove them in their mouth as fast as they can. Maybe they hit the drive-thru and order the triple burger, extra-large fries, gigantic pop and sweet dessert to top it all off.

The reason why diet plans don't work is because they most likely don't fit your lifestyle, your likes and dislikes. They fail to take into account the emotional core issues that trigger over-eating. Additionally, they fail to meet the body's nutritional wants, needs and desires, and they eliminate or greatly restrict all your favourite food items which ultimately leaves you feeling deprived. Feeling deprived is never a good thing! When this happens your body responds like a spoiled child and it throws a tantrum, and you are almost helpless to stop the rage.

Traditional restricted *"diets"* designed to reduce caloric intake are not built for real life, they are not sustainable and they teach you very little about your body's nutritional needs.

If you want to lose weight then you have to consider maybe, just maybe, the food you are consuming isn't working in the best interest of your body's needs. Maybe it's the wrong formula, the wrong stuff, too much of one thing, too little of another. Consider that your current diet is out of balance.

Chances are you are starving your body in one regard and stuffing it in another.

Your body deserves more than this. It wants variety and tasty pleasure, it needs life-giving vitamins and nutrients, and it desires joyful deliciousness. It also wants to move easily with strength and vitality. It wants to be free and alive and the only way to get there is to make changes that will fuel it for success. There is no way around it.

You can't keep eating the way you are while also depriving yourself of the joy of movement and expect that your weight or energy levels are going to change. It's not going to happen. You can wish for it, hope for it, think about it, but it's not going to happen unless you take positive, healthy steps in the direction of your goal.

Start your journey by taking a good look at the foods you are currently eating: be honest. Are you eating too many simple carbohydrates like I was? Are you getting enough protein like I wasn't? Do you eat healthy fat every day? I know I certainly wasn't, I stayed clear of fats like avocado, and nuts – way too many calories and not filling!

Whoa, what a mistake that was!

If you are anything like me you will most likely need to change not only what you eat and how much, but, you will also need to rethink some of your food beliefs. I now know that healthy fat is essential for the proper function of my body and I now eat it every day.

Our bodies are miraculous biological machines needing proper fuel and care. So make a decision to put only the best fuel into your machine. Choose quality over quantity and you will not go wrong.

When I grocery shop I buy organic products as much as possible while working within my budget and what is available. I believe that organic products are higher quality: I believe them to be free from harmful sprays, chemicals and pesticides. I am not interested in putting these harmful products in my body (or on my body for that matter), so I limit my exposure to them.

I also believe in buying products that are grown and made locally. For so many reasons I believe this to be a better choice for our bodies and for our environment. I once heard someone speak about the importance of buying honey from a producer in your own local area because the bees know what your local environment is in need of and so the bees will produce the honey accordingly. This fascinates me; Mother Nature in general fascinates me.

I grow a lot of my own vegetables in my backyard garden. I love doing this. I love watching the seeds sprout out of the ground. I love watching the plants bloom. I love seeing the bees busy pollinating the plants. I love watching the vegetables grow from tiny specs to edible delicious food. I love how garden fresh vegetables taste and how good I feel after eating them.

It also blows my mind how much food I can grow for so little. One spring I decided to save the seeds from an organic butternut squash that I had purchased. I dried the seeds and planted about six of them in my garden.

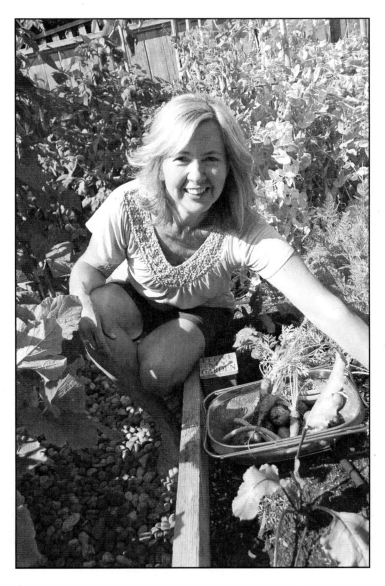

In my garden. I love growing my own vegetables.

I was curious if the seeds would sprout. Much to my amazement, not only did they sprout, but they produced at least 12 new gorgeous and delicious butternut squash. I got so much food, all from that one original squash. Talk about value! I have since done the same thing with spaghetti squash and cantaloupe seeds as well as potatoes and yams. What a joy!

The point here is not to grow your own vegetables, obviously that is not feasible for many people. What is feasible though is for you to start to choose foods that are of a higher quality, foods grown organically, made locally and that will fuel and nourish the cells of your body. Think in terms of eating food from the earth not from a factory. This makes sense to me on so many levels. Not only will you taste the difference but your body will feel the difference.

My body is much happier when I feed it this way and I know yours will be too. The amazing thing is that once I started to fuel my body with nutritious food I automatically ate less – it's true! Real, wholesome food from the earth provides your body with so much goodness that it will be satisfied and fulfilled.

Don't get me wrong, eating less food might be something you need to do, but the good news is that you don't have to spend too much of your time and energy focusing on cutting back on the quantity of food you are consuming. Instead, focus your time and energy on the quality of food you are eating and the quantity will take care of itself. Remember, if you fill your body with food that lacks the required nutrients, it will never be satisfied, it will constantly be craving more and it will not provide you with the energy you need to get through your day with ease and happiness.

On the other hand, if you fuel your body with real, fresh, natural, colourful whole food, your engine will be super-charged and you will be able to take on your day with vigour and enthusiasm. Give your body the best that you can, fill it with goodness and watch as your body comes alive.

Right now I can hear many of you say that organic foods cost too much or that they cost more than non-organic. Although this may be true in some cases, it is not true in all cases. Check the prices. On several occasions I have actually found organic fruits and vegetables to be less expensive than their nonorganic counterparts. Compare the prices, look for sales, or check out farmers markets. Better yet, buy a package of organic seeds, put them in some dirt and watch them multiply. You will be blown away by how much food you can produce from your initial $4.00 seed investment. If you live in an apartment and don't have access to a plot of land, no problem: put the seeds in a pot and watch magic happen. Many varieties of vegetables grow really well in pots.

I also regularly buy a two-pack of organic chicken from Costco. They usually cost around $36.00, or $18.00 per chicken. I usually roast the chicken for dinner one night, serving it with mashed potatoes and two to three vegetables. The following day we make chicken sandwiches or put cut-up chicken in a salad. I usually finish off the remaining chicken by making chicken enchiladas the following night. I always freeze the bones so that I can use them later to make my own stock. Not only do I save the chicken bones, but I also save vegetable scraps. Once I get a full bag of veggie scraps and bones, I put them in my slow cooker and fill it with water. I let it cook on low for about eight hours. The resulting stock is rich, nutritious and makes a great base for homemade soup.

The initial $36.00 cost for the two organic chickens gave us several meals and several litres of delicious stock! You can't go wrong. These days, on the rare occasion that our family of three eats at a fast-food restaurant, the cost is around $36.00 and we get one crappy meal each! It's a no-brainer which investment is the better deal!

Start to think of food as your friend; someone you enjoy spending time with. It should be nurturing and supportive in all the best and most loving of ways. I love food. I love eating and I eat a lot. But the difference now is in the quality of the food I eat. This for me was the biggest change I made.

Today I eat totally different than I did when I was overweight, lethargic and on the verge of major health issues. I eat better and therefore I feel better.

I have no doubt in my mind that when you start to experiment with new healthy food choices that your body will wake up and rejoice at the love you are showing it.

Making changes does not have to be an overwhelming, daunting experience. Instead, make it an exciting journey. Don't try to change everything at once. Instead, take your time and have fun; experiment, play with your food, try new things. Make it a game to try a new food or a new recipe every few days. The internet is full of exciting, delicious and healthy recipes. Don't be overwhelmed. Pick one recipe per week that is loaded with nutrient rich foods, and then make it. Pay special attention to how you feel after eating this meal. Then make another new, healthy recipe the next week.

It really is exciting to eat something that you have never eaten before and discover that you really like it. It's even more exciting when you start playing around with recipes and come up with something really good and your family looks at you in disbelief that you actually made this because it tastes delicious and you know that it is also good for them too. These are the moments of pride and progression when we celebrate our victories. These victories fuel us and encourage us to try other new recipes or other new foods. It is a journey of discovery and it can be a lot of fun!

The more I researched "new-to-me" foods and new recipes, the more astonished I was. Discovering recipes like "Quinoa Chocolate Cake" "Black Bean Brownies", and "Cauliflower Pizza Crust" opened a flood gate of never-ending healthier alternatives.

We just need to change our thoughts and open our minds and new ideas will pour in. But, we have to be willing and then we have to watch and listen to suggestions and then we have to take a step forward. With desire, dedication, practice and persistence you can build a new, healthy lifestyle and hopefully you will never go hungry again.

I am so grateful that I no longer have to be on the roller coaster ride of diets. I am so thankful that I now understand how food is fuel for my body. I am so happy that I now know how to control my food cravings and control my blood sugar levels through balanced, delicious, healthy eating. Mostly, I feel joy in sharing what I have learned. Thank you for sticking with me so far.

Chapter 5

What I Ate and How I Made the Changes

This chapter further explains some of the changes I made to my diet and why I made the changes. My goal was to improve my health so I could live a more active, vibrant life. I had no choice but to change my relationship with food which meant educating myself on what food was. I adopted a new attitude that food was fuel and if I was going to eat something I asked myself over and over:

- "What is the purpose of this food?"
- "Would a healthy person eat this?"
- "How will I feel after I eat this?"
- "Will this food sustain me and nourish me?"
- "Is this meal balanced and complete?"

Asking these questions set me up for success. By saying *"yes"* to healthy choices and *"no"* to unhealthy choices I slowly started to feel and see changes in my body. Remember, I made these changes one at a time. I will begin to explain the changes I made by starting with the changes I made to my breakfasts.

Breakfast

When I was young I grew up eating boxed cereal and toast for breakfast (wheat, refined sugars and preservatives). Sometimes we had a special treat of toaster pastries or pancakes made from a boxed mix (more wheat, refined sugar and preservatives). Occasionally we had grapefruit, which we sprinkled with sugar. Fruit was not a staple in the morning; fruit was reserved for special occasions where we might have a fruit salad (from a can), usually with an imitation whipped cream on top, which I despised. On cold winter days we had oatmeal or cream of wheat with brown sugar on top (more wheat, more sugar). Breakfast was breakfast and I never really questioned what I ate, I just ate it because that is what was put in front of me.

As I got older, I introduced eggs and toast, yogurt (flavoured) and on special occasions: eggs benedict covered in hollandaise sauce. But, for the most part the only breakfast items I took into my adulthood from my childhood were cereal and toast. Of course, in my adulthood, I did eat the *"healthier"* fortified, whole wheat, sugar-free, fat-free, enriched cereals!! In other words: processed, preserved, simple carbs in a box!

Changing what I ate for breakfast was a very slow and unintentional process. It came about because I finally started to pay attention to how I felt after I ate breakfast in the morning. I discovered that cereal and toast did not sustain me, however, oatmeal did. Oatmeal became a very important food choice on my journey.

Oatmeal

As a kid oatmeal was never my favourite breakfast. I never really liked the texture and I never liked all the brown sugar that was customary in our family to sprinkle on top. But, oatmeal was hardy and *"would stick to my ribs on a cold winter day,"* so I reluctantly ate it when it was placed in front of me.

As an adult I could choose to eat it or not, and mostly I chose not to eat it. However, as I started my healthy lifestyle journey I came across lots of information on the health benefits of oats. Simply put, oats contain protein, carbohydrates and fat, as well as many important vitamins and minerals. They are also rich in fibre and antioxidants. Eating oats sounded like a healthy food choice, so I decided to give oats another try.

But first I had to learn the differences between the different types of oats. What I learned was that **steel-cut oats** and **old-fashioned oats** take longer to absorb and digest meaning they offer a steady flow of energy for the body. **Quick oats** on the other hand are more refined and are quickly absorbed into the body meaning that the resulting energy is short-lived. Since I wanted an even flow of energy and not a burst of energy, I chose to eat old-fashioned oats. I do sometimes eat steel-cut oats, but I find they take much longer to cook and so I prefer old-fashioned or large flake oats.

Next, I had to come up with a replacement for the brown sugar so I started to eat my oatmeal with fruit, all kinds of fruit: blueberries, strawberries, bananas, peaches, and apples and cinnamon. Sometimes I added a teaspoon of organic jam. Then I started to sprinkle hemp seeds, flax seeds and slivered toasted almonds or walnuts on top. Eating oatmeal this way was delicious and fulfilling and most importantly I realized that I did not experience the blood sugar crashes that I did when I ate cereal and toast.

On my oatmeal journey I came across recipes for *overnight oats.* This came in particularly handy when I was getting up at 5:30 am to catch a 7:00 am train into Vancouver to work. The first few times I made overnight oats I followed the recipes that I found online precisely, including making them and storing them in cute little mason jars! Seriously, a cute idea but I always made a mess getting all the ingredients in and out of the narrow opening. I found the mason jars to be very unpractical, so I made the grand decision to ditch the mason jars and I started to make my overnight oats in wide mouth containers with snap on lids. This worked out much better for me. I could eat my oats on the train without losing a spoonful of oats down the front of my shirt, and I think they tasted just as good in a more practical container.

The other thing that I discovered about overnight oats is that you don't have to soak them overnight! I now often throw the oats in a bowl with some flax seeds, hemp seeds, chia seeds, frozen fruit and almond milk. I let it sit on the counter for 30-60 minutes or so and as the fruit unthaws, the oats soften and when I am ready to eat, the oats are ready for me. It works out perfectly. I now enjoy oatmeal on a regular basis; it fuels my body with nutrients and keeps my blood sugars consistent, which is such a wonderful feeling.

As you begin to experiment with recipes, don't be afraid to make changes that suit you and your lifestyle, your likes and your dislikes. For me, I will never eat my oatmeal out of a mason jar and I will never again sprinkle it with brown sugar.

Greek Yogurt

Greek yogurt became one of my best friends early on in my journey. In my past I had often eaten yogurt but mostly flavoured yogurt. Once I started to pay closer attention to labels I noticed how little protein and how much sugar (simple carbohydrate – which converts to fat) there is in flavoured yogurt. I read and discovered that Greek yogurt is much higher in protein so I made the switch to unflavoured Greek yogurt. Now let me also say that I can feel my cheeks puckering up at the thought of straight up Greek yogurt! In my opinion it is very tart and so, for me, I needed to sweeten it up a little. I now usually eat my Greek yogurt with cut-up fruit, flax seeds, hemp seeds, almond slices and a heaping teaspoon of organic blueberry or raspberry jam. It is a balanced breakfast of protein, carbohydrates and healthy fat. The balanced combination of macronutrients fuels the cells of my body with everything they need to perform their tasks. Additionally, the balanced nutrients prevent my blood sugar levels from spiking and crashing. What this means is that I am less likely to experience the *'shaky, starving'* sensation that often sees me reaching for quick-fix unhealthy foods.

Greek yogurt played a very important role in my weight loss journey. I ate it regularly; it was convenient, high in protein, fast, could be eaten in a variety of ways and was always filling and satisfying. But, I also started to learn about the less desirable side of Greek yogurt and dairy products in general. Dairy products are acidic to our body's systems. What this means is that when we ingest too many acidic foods the PH levels in our bodies can be affected. Our bodies operate most efficiently with a balanced PH level. When our internal systems are too acidic we open the doors and invite all kinds of health problems in. Much is written about the health benefits of consuming neutral or alkaline foods and avoiding acidic foods. I am far from an expert in this field so I will just share that these facts resonate with me and so as time goes on and I learn more about how foods affect our bodies, I find that I am naturally eating less Greek yogurt for breakfast and I am drawn to eating more vegetables for breakfast.

I believe that it is in the best interest of my body to reduce the amounts of acidic foods that I eat. Don't get me wrong, I still eat dairy products like Greek yogurt, cheese, butter and sour cream, but I have cut down and will continue to do so. Here are some of the ways I have reduced my consumption of dairy products:

- I rarely drink cow's milk now; in its place I use almond 'milk'.
- I often swap out butter for coconut oil in several of my recipes.
- I have been experimenting with nutritional yeast as a cheese flavoured substitute in sauces and soups.

Please don't misunderstand me; I am not advocating that you eliminate dairy products from your diet. What I am suggesting is that you do some research and make changes that make sense to you. I am also suggesting that you eat a variety of foods, continue to experiment and learn to listen to your body.

There are days that my body wants Greek yogurt for breakfast and so that is what I give it. And, every couple of months or so I get a craving for a glass of cold milk and so I have one and it tastes great. Also, I love cheese and can't imagine my life without it, but, I believe that there are ways to cut down on the amount of cheese I eat without feeling deprived. In addition, when I do choose dairy products, I try to purchase organic as much as possible. I think it's a better choice for my body.

I love trying new things and testing recipes to see if I can make them healthier. It is fun and interesting to me and I never get bored. Not all recipes are keepers but many are.

When you look at your own breakfast food choices, are there things that you could change? Are there items that you can eliminate, alter, or substitute that will make your meal less acidic, more balanced and complete with protein, healthy carbohydrates and essential fats?

Veggies for Breakfast

I remember the first time I saw someone eat a salad for breakfast, I was dumbfounded! I thought: *"You can't eat a salad for breakfast! That makes no sense! Salad is for lunch or dinner, not for breakfast!"* It was an obscure concept. But, then I thought about a trip I had made to Turkey several years earlier. They ate veggies for breakfast. I remember well; every single breakfast was the same, tomatoes, cucumbers, olives and bread. Since I didn't like tomatoes and olives, I survived by eating the cucumbers and bread.

Fast forward to my current journey and I realize now that introducing vegetables into my breakfast routine was probably one of the healthiest, smartest decisions I could have made. No, I did not start by eating a salad for breakfast. (Actually, to this day, I have never had a salad for breakfast.) I started adding vegetables to my breakfast by including them in my morning smoothie.

One morning I took a leap of faith and decided to throw the leftover mashed yams from dinner the night before into my morning smoothie! It worked out great. The yams added thickness, colour and nutrition to my smoothie and that was a good thing. This positive experience nudged me forward and I experimented with adding all types of veggies to my smoothie. I now add veggies of some sort to almost all my smoothies including: kale, spinach, cucumbers, squash, lettuce, beets, yams, carrots and broccoli. I balance out the flavours by adding mint, cocoa and fruits like bananas, blueberries, pineapple, pears, peaches, strawberries, mango and avocado. The list goes on. I do have a couple of smoothie recipes that I follow, but, mostly I just throw in whatever I have on hand and if it tastes weird I add more banana or blueberries. That usually does the trick! Adding vegetables to your morning smoothie is a great way to get more vegetables into your body in a fast, easy, delicious and nutritious way.

The next step in my desire to add more vegetables into my breakfast again came quite by accident. One day I was making scrambled eggs and decided to throw in some leftover roasted veggies that were in my fridge. Wham! That was a good idea, so along with all the protein in the eggs I was now adding lots of complex carbohydrates. There is no magic recipe; just scramble up the eggs and throw in whatever precooked vegetables that you have in your fridge which could include yams, cauliflower, potatoes, carrots, corn, beans, asparagus, broccoli, spinach or kale. To add some healthy fat you can scramble your eggs in olive oil, sprinkle with hemp seeds, or serve the eggs with a piece of avocado. Now you have a perfectly balanced meal that will fuel your body for hours to come.

One of my other favourite ways to enjoy vegetables at breakfast came about because I needed to find a healthy alternative to eggs benedict. The first thing that I needed to figure out was what to use in place of the English muffin. I came across a recipe for yam waffles. I thought *that sounds good.* So I tried the recipe and it was good, but I decided to modify it and add a few things and then I tried it again. I probably changed the original recipe four or five times until I came up with my version of healthy yam waffles. I top the waffles with spinach, basted or poached eggs, avocado and a drizzle of maple syrup. I know this is not a replacement for eggs benedict but it is a special treat that takes a little extra time to prepare and it tastes delicious and decadent. I love the combination of sweet and savoury. My body feels completely nourished after eating this veggie packed breakfast. My yam waffle recipe is on page 204.

Eating veggies for breakfast alongside a serving of protein and healthy fats will fuel your body and provide an even source of energy. In other words, your blood sugar levels will remain constant throughout the morning and you will not experience those nasty mid-morning hunger pains. Vegetables will fill your body with so much goodness, so many nutrients, lots of fibre and believe me they are tasty. I wouldn't eat them if they weren't. After eating a breakfast loaded with vegetables I can literally get on with my day and not even think about food for a few hours: my body is truly satisfied and fulfilled.

Adding vegetables to my morning breakfast routine was a game changer, and one of the smartest changes I made on my wellness journey.

So, go ahead, shake things up. Try eating vegetables for breakfast. You might not be ready to dive in and eat a salad for breakfast, I don't blame you, I'm not there yet either. But, do your body a favour and start experimenting with the endless ways you can incorporate vegetables into your breakfast. Step outside the box, try new things. You might not throw out your boxed cereals, toast and bagels right away, and that's okay. But, with persistence you will soon find that eating veggies for breakfast might help change your life. Your body will be loaded with lots of life-giving fuel. You will have more energy to perform your daily tasks. You will feel better, look better and sleep better. At least that's what happened for me.

Snacking

I am a huge fan of snacking. I can honestly say that I believe snacking is a huge reason that I have been successful on my weight loss journey. What would life be without snacks? Wonderful little breaks in the day to sit and indulge. Remember as a child sitting down to milk and cookies? How good was that? If your mom let you, maybe you dipped your cookies in your milk. Snacking is important and necessary and I snack every day; morning, afternoon, and night.

Snacking gives you a mental break in your day to day grind and it should be used as a time to refuel your body and give your mind a necessary break. But, before you reach for the bag of chips or chocolate bar thinking, *"But you said I could and should snack!"* let's be clear that junk food snacking is not fuelling your body for success.

These snacks may be quick, easy, tasty, momentarily satisfying and have saved many a person, including myself, from *starving to death*! But, don't be fooled by the false promises that these snacks make. They may fill your belly momentarily but that is where the *benefits* end! Most of these convenient snacks so readily available at grocery stores, gas stations, vending machines and convenience stores are not good for you! They have no nutritional value, they are full of unhealthy fats, sugar, preservatives and chemicals designed to make you addicted to them.

The companies who make these products do not care about you; they don't care about your health, your well-being or your goals. They care about one thing and one thing only, and that is profit!

I must confess that there are times that I succumb to their lure and promises of deliciousness. There are times when I am so hungry, I am unprepared, and I cave! I stop off at a convenience store and pick up some crappy snack, even though the healthy, rational side of my brain is whispering at me, *"Don't do it Rhonda."* The other part of my brain that has been taken over by the ravenous bull is yelling, *"YES! YES! YES!"* and I eat the snack and immediately feel gross.

NO! NO! NO! These are not the types of snacks I am talking about. The types of snacks I am talking about are made from real food, and the best snacks are the ones that contain protein, carbohydrates and healthy fat. Why? Because the right combination of these macronutrients will fuel your body's needs. Snacks heavy in simple carbohydrates will mess with your body's function and you will suffer, and why would you want to do that?

I have a number of snacks that I like to eat, but my two favourite snacks are almonds and homemade muffins. Let me explain:

Almonds

One of my favourite snacks is almonds. Yes, almonds! These babies are my best friend. I carry a little jar of almonds with me all the time. I know what you are thinking: *"But, almonds are full of fat!"* Yes, you are correct, but it's the **HEALTHY FAT,** people! Our bodies need healthy fat. It is vital for the proper functioning of our cells. Healthy fat helps protect our heart, brain and other vital organs. Healthy fat aids in the absorption of vitamins and is vital for the proper functioning of the immune system. Not having enough healthy fat in your body can actually lead to weakened immune systems, organ damage and can create cravings for fat (usually unhealthy fat). People....you need to hear this:

Healthy fat is vital to your health: eat it today and every day!

A small handful of almonds contain protein, healthy fat, and a small amount of carbohydrates and fibre. I eat almonds often as a mid-morning or afternoon snack. When paired with an apple, this is the perfect snack to satisfy my body's need for nourishment. I love spreading almond butter on apple slices; this is so delicious and nourishing. The almonds and apples work together to stabilize my blood sugar levels leaving me satisfied and fulfilled. I will often eat a handful of almonds before going out for dinner. I do this so that I don't arrive at the restaurant starving and then proceed to wolf down the bread or buns that are often presented at the start of the meal. I also put almonds in my yogurt or oatmeal in the morning. I grind almonds up into flour which I use in my muffins and cookies. I carry almonds with me all the time because when I am out doing errands and I feel the hunger pangs come up, I can eat a few almonds and right away I feel better. There is something magical in those little crunchy nuts! I love how they work in my body; so simple and so easy. If you haven't gotten to know almonds yet I urge you to try them. Almonds are a good friend to have and will treat your body with lots of love and respect.

Obviously, there are people who are allergic to almonds. If you are one of those people then you will have to experiment with other handy nourishing snacks to find the one that you can easily carry with you, one that you can depend upon to give you a quick, nutritional boost when you need it.

Muffins – My Other Favourite Snack

I am going to start this part of the chapter by saying: I LOVE MUFFINS! Many years ago a friend and I had a routine: at least three times a week we got together early in the morning for a workout, and then we headed out for a coffee, a bowl of French vanilla yogurt and a muffin. We did this for at least a couple of years. I really don't remember losing any weight with all that working out, but I do remember the muffins. They were so good, crunchy on top, moist and delicious inside. I would dip my muffin in the yogurt and my mouth would do a happy dance. These were good days of guilt-free eating: I had worked out so I could easily enjoy the muffin without regret.

Eventually, our routine changed. I moved to a new city and so no longer could we meet for our early morning workouts, coffee and muffins. However, my love of coffee and muffins in the morning had become a routine that continued for years until I finally made the connection between wheat and my zigzagging blood sugar levels. I finally realized that within two hours of eating a muffin, I was starving again. I concluded that I was going to have to say goodbye to muffins. After all, these muffins were full of wheat and sugar and most likely unhealthy fat. I knew that these muffins were not good for me and did not nourish my body.

But, my love of muffins stayed with me. Not eating them made me feel deprived and I didn't like that feeling so I wondered how I could make a *healthy muffin*, one without wheat and sugar and unhealthy fat.

So, I started to research **'healthy muffins'**, **'wheat alternatives'** and **'sugar substitutions'** online. What I discovered is that there are countless recipes for healthy muffins using all types of flour alternatives and sugar replacements. I learned that not all flours and sugar are created equal. In particular, I learned that the traditional, commercial brands of flour and sugar are produced to yield the highest volume for the least amount of money which, of course, increases profits for the producers and manufacturers. When I educated myself about what our flour and sugar go through before they end up on our grocery shelf I was stunned and appalled. How is this allowed to happen? I guess the answer is: money!

But, what can I, the consumer, do about it? I can make new choices and so that is what I did. I started to look for healthier options for traditional flour and refined sugar. What I discovered was that there are several healthy options available, and so, I started to experiment. In my baking, I now replace regular, old white or whole wheat flour with: spelt flour, buckwheat flour, oat flour, almond flour, flaxseed meal, and coconut flour. (A word of caution about coconut flour: you cannot swap out regular flour for coconut flour because it is about four times more absorbent. I learned that the hard way.)

I also ditched the refined white sugar that I had been using my whole life and replaced it with organic palm sugar and organic cane sugar. Additionally, sometimes I use honey, maple syrup, dates or bananas as a sweetener in my recipes. These sweeteners are less processed or come straight from nature. Our bodies know how to use them, they are easily digested.

These healthier alternative flours and sugars are readily available in the health food section of most major grocery stores and recently I have found some of them at Costco. As consumers we do have the power to make change based on our choices. Choose wisely and not only will you be helping to change the food industry, but you will also be making major changes to the health of your body.

As I experimented and played around with lots of recipes I eventually came up with a few muffin recipes that were not only delicious and satisfying but they were also packed with protein, healthy fats and carbohydrates.

I can now enjoy eating muffins again knowing that my homemade muffins will nourish my body, control my blood sugar level, eliminate cravings and leave me feeling very satisfied. On page 218 I share one of my favourite recipes that I created: Chocolate Zucchini Quinoa Muffins. I often double the recipe because my sister Dianne says, *"Why spend the time making 12 muffins when you can just as easily make 24."* Thanks for the tip, sis!

Planning healthy, nourishing, tasty, well-balanced snacks was a huge part of my successful weight loss. The possibilities are endless. Here is a list of some of my go-to snacks:

- A piece of fruit and a few almonds (10-12)
- Healthy homemade muffins
- Cut-up veggies with hummus or tzatziki
- Crispy corn thin cakes with nut butter, egg salad, or cheese
- Apples or banana with nut or seed butter
- Rice crackers, cheese and jalapeño jelly
- Popcorn
- Grapes and cheese
- Homemade energy balls or granola bars
- Homemade cookies (always healthy and balanced)
- Smoothie
- Homemade "ice cream" (frozen fruit in a blender)

Snacking is good, snacking is wonderful. Rethink what you snack on. Avoid the pre-packaged 100 calorie snacks; they are void of nutrition, do nothing for your body and the only person they benefit are the people who are lining their pockets from the sale of these useless empty 'snacks.' Eat real food at snack time. Eat protein, healthy fat and carbohydrates. Drink lots of water or herbal tea. Fuel your body for success. Really think about your food. How will it serve you? Will it satisfy your taste buds or will it also send life-giving nutrients to all the cells of your body. Choose your snacks with these thoughts in mind. You will feel amazing!

Happy, healthy snacking!

Pizza

Who doesn't love pizza? In our house it is a regular at least once every couple of weeks. Sometimes we order in but mostly we make our own pizzas at home because we can make them healthier and we can each personalize our pizzas with all our favourite toppings. Because of my decision to eliminate wheat, I needed to look at my options for a wheat-free pizza crust. At the time there was buzz on social media about cauliflower pizza crust. Awesome! I selected one of the recipes I found online and then proceeded to make the crust as per the directions. I really liked this *pizza crust*. The flavour to me was awesome. But, there were some problems with this crust. First, the crust didn't hold together (it wasn't very crusty), second, it was quite time consuming to make, and third, I couldn't get my family to eat it! The first problem was solved when an acquaintance of mine suggested that I add cooked quinoa to the crust mixture before cooking it. She said that's what she did and it worked great. So, I gave it a try and it worked; at least for the most part the crust stayed together. I love the flavour of this crust, it is so versatile. I always make a big batch and freeze them so I can quickly pop one in the toaster to use under poached eggs, or I can make myself a healthy pizza, or I love, love, love making a grilled cheese '*sandwich*' with them.

However, my family was not keen on this version of pizza crust, so back to the internet I went in search of inspiration. I came across a recipe from www.simplyquinoa.com which used quinoa that had been soaked in water as the base for the recipe. I was intrigued, so I went to work experimenting with the recipe. I changed the measurements, added a couple for ingredients and I changed the cooking time. Jackpot! I came up with a winner. This pizza crust is delicious, holds together perfectly, is crunchy and best of all, my family will eat it.

I share my two pizza crust recipes on pages 212 to 213.

You may be wondering why all the fuss over pizza. The answer is simple, because I love pizza and I don't want to give it up. But, I need pizza that is delicious and nutritious. Quinoa again, is a complete protein, so when combined with all the healthy complex carbohydrate toppings (spinach, peppers, mushrooms, artichoke hearts, pineapple) and healthy fats (pesto and olives), this pizza will give my body all the essential nutrients it needs. It will fill my mouth with the deliciousness it wants and the combination of crunchy, creamy, tangy, sweet textures will fill its desires. It's a perfect combination and my body is much happier when I feed it this pizza than when I feed it pizza that we order in. And yes, I still put cheese on my pizza because I love it that way!

Don't get me wrong, we still sometimes order in pizza because I really need a night off from cooking. It is great to be at the point in my wellness journey that I can eat gooey restaurant pizza and not worry too much about it. Although I am not feeding my body the best at that meal, I enjoy the pizza and move on to the next healthy meal after that.

I am not asking you to give up pizza, but, I am suggesting that it is possible to make nutritious, homemade pizza that also tastes amazing.

Changing our old ways is the goal but, it doesn't need to be done overnight. Enjoy the process and with each victory you will gain confidence and you will begin to find new ways that work better for your body. You will find new things to eat that you enjoy even more than the old standbys. The possibilities are endless. There is a whole new world of tastes just waiting for you to discover.

Pasta

Oh pasta, beautiful pasta, how I love you… well, let me rephrase that. I used to love you until I realized that you were actually not good for me. My taste buds might like you but my insides don't. So, I had no choice but to change up my favourite pasta dishes. I had to say goodbye to wheat-based pasta.

Firstly, I discovered **ramen noodles**. No, I am not talking about the ramen noodles that come with the salty, flavour packages. I am talking about ramen noodles made from organic millet and brown rice. The brand that I buy is gluten free, vegan, high in protein and fibre and takes only four minutes to cook. I love to serve these noodles tossed together with cooked vegetables, pesto and avocado. Sometimes I add chunks of cooked chicken or prawns. This meal is quick, creamy and delicious and fuels my body with all kinds of goodness.

Although there is no exact recipe, I share how I make it on page 215.

Lasagne: Gone are the days of traditional lasagne. I just can't eat it anymore. It bloats me and leaves me feeling stuffed. These days I make a vegetable-layered lasagne using zucchini strips, red peppers, spinach, sundried tomatoes, quinoa, pesto, feta cheese and tomato sauce. No, it's not the same as traditional lasagne: it's better.

Spaghetti and Meat Sauce: Who doesn't love spaghetti and meat sauce? It's a staple and a quick go-to meal. However, when I stopped eating wheat I had to find an alternative for the noodles. I also decided that I wanted to add more vegetables to the meat sauce. Today my spaghetti and meat sauce is never the same twice. I use what I have. Sometimes I add pureed carrots or squash to the meat sauce. Sometimes I add mushrooms or peppers and for sure I add lots of pureed tomatoes. For noodles: sometimes I use ramen noodles, sometimes I use rice noodles, but, most often I use spaghetti squash. I feel good loading up on vegetables and I always skip on the garlic toast. Do I feel deprived? Absolutely not. Actually, I feel bad for people who deprive their bodies of the benefits of loads of vegetables and instead stuff it with so many simple carbs. It just isn't a choice anymore; I know what works for my body.

I share my tips for making a healthier version of spaghetti and meat sauce on page 214.

Mac and Cheese: One should not live life without once in a while indulging in a delicious and creamy bowl of mac and cheese. So, once again I began my search for a perfectly delicious, creamy recipe that was also wheat-free and loaded with vegetables. Vegetables in mac and cheese you ask? Yes. I don't know where I found my original recipe but there are lots of them online. The trick is to add butternut squash puree to the cheese mixture and then double up on vegetables by adding in broccoli or peas as well. To make my mac and cheese wheat-free, I use organic, brown rice, macaroni noodles. This meal is the real deal: creamy comfort food at its best and it is also good for you! Plus, my son loves it too (minus the peas)! Do some research, look for "Butternut Squash Mac and Cheese" online and give one of the recipes a try. You can even take this idea one step further by using nutritional yeast in place of some or all of the cheese in the sauce. I most often use part nutritional yeast and part cheese because I love cheese and to me nothing beats the flavour. This way I get the flavour but also all the goodness of the nutritional yeast. What could be better?

I hope that you like some of my pasta ideas. Pasta is a big deal in our culture, unfortunately I believe that our wheat has been modified so much that our bodies barely recognize it as something it can use. It seems that it has been stripped of all the original goodness and instead, it just turns quickly into sugar in our systems and then to fat. We have to pay attention. We have to look for healthier options: options that fuel and serve our bodies. No one is expected to live life without these classical favourites. It is time however to update old recipes using higher quality ingredients that fuel and protect the cells in our body. It works for me! My body is healthier, stronger and I have a lot more energy. Real food works!

Desserts

Cake

A while back a friend of mine was telling me about the plans she had made for a big family birthday party to celebrate her daughter's 14th birthday. She was telling me about all the prep work she had done and the wonderful cupcakes she lovingly made for her daughter. They were cream filled and topped with buttercream icing. She was also telling me about how awful she was feeling that afternoon because she had eaten another one of those delicious cupcakes for her afternoon coffee break. I commented simply by saying that she could have made a healthier version cupcake that wouldn't make her feel so awful. She said, *"But, I wouldn't do that for a 14-year-old!"* Of course what she meant was that 'healthy' in her mind wasn't congruous to a delicious birthday cake for her beautiful daughter.

But, here lies the problem: most of the ingredients that go into a traditional birthday cake are not ingredients that the body can use and is starving for. I am guessing that the number one ingredient in the cake was flour, followed by sugar, and then probably butter or oil or shortening of some type: all ingredients that don't serve the body. Then my poor friend wondered why she felt like crap. The reality is, no matter how much love you put into the cake it isn't going to change the ingredients.

I am here to tell you that you can make a healthy, delicious, life-giving cake befitting any celebration.

> *Finding healthy substitutes is one of the main things I did to help me on my weight loss journey. I didn't want to give up taste and pleasure, but I did want to give up useless, harmful ingredients that did not serve my body.*

One of the first healthy cakes I made was a quinoa chocolate cake. I heard about the cake from a friend of mine. She told me that the recipe called for cooked quinoa in the place of flour. *Really?* I was intrigued, so I looked up the recipe online and sure enough there it was. The first cake I made was actually kind of exciting and it turned out great. My family liked it and I felt much better about serving this to my family than serving them a previous chocolate cake recipe that I had from a lifetime ago that had all the usual ingredients in it. In this recipe, cooked quinoa was used in the place of flour. What a brilliant idea! You may ask, *"What does quinoa have to do with it?"* Quinoa is considered a super-food: it is a complete protein meaning it has all the essential amino acids. It is also a complex carbohydrate and is chock-full of vitamins and minerals and antioxidants. So, in combination with the other carbohydrates and fats in the recipe, it is actually a fairly balanced recipe. What I didn't like about the recipe was that it still had a fair amount of sugar. So, I went about experimenting with natural, healthier alternatives for the sugar. In the end I replaced the sugar with coconut palm sugar. It processes in the blood slower and therefore does not spike my blood sugar level the way regular, refined white sugar does. This makes me feel better.

After the quinoa chocolate cake recipe, I heard from another source about black bean brownies. *What?* Okay, this I had to try, so back to Google I went and there it was: a recipe for Black Bean Brownies. I made it and my family gobbled them down (not knowing that they contained black beans). I made them again, and they gobbled them down again. The third time I made them my son came into the kitchen and looked in the food processor and said, *"Ewe! I'm not eating that!"* I tried to reassure him that he would love them because he had loved them when I made them before. He declared, *"No way!"* and unfortunately never ate them again. So my advice: if you have kids who are picky eaters, you might not want them to know what those goodies are made of.

After this experience I decided that I needed a new chocolate cake recipe, so once again I went back to my computer hunting for inspirational recipes. I tried a few; some were great, some not so much. I liked the idea of adding avocado to my chocolate cake, but the recipes I tried were disappointing to me. What did I do? I made my own recipe. Yes, it contains black beans (protein and fibre) and avocado (healthy fat and fibre), but this recipe is delicious! This is my favourite. It is moist, healthy, and balanced. Actually, it is more of a brownie than a cake. But, it is delicious; especially when topped with a creamy topping I make and served with a side of fresh berries.

I have served this brownie to company with rave reviews and they all want the recipe. My husband loves this brownie and yes, he knows it has black beans in it. My son, well, he is coming around!

You can find the recipes for my chocolate brownie and creamy topping on pages 219 - 221.

Chocolate cake, brownies and cookies are all part of what makes life so sweet. Most standard diets eliminate these sweet indulgences. But, how are we supposed to live on a diet that restricts the pleasure of the delectable baked goodies. It's not realistic. We absolutely need to be able to enjoy these desserts. Furthermore, we should never feel guilty and we should never apologize for enjoying these delicious moments that celebrate life and love.

On my journey I have chosen to include desserts and baked goodies because I don't want to live my life without them. What I did was find recipes that used healthier ingredients, less sugar, less unhealthy fat, were mostly wheat free and have some protein to balance out the carbs. I changed a lot of my old recipes and I did a lot of experimenting. I had to throw out some of my experiments because they were not edible. I learned the hard way that you cannot substitute coconut flour for regular wheat flour: those cookies ended up in the garbage, lesson learned. I also learned the hard way that my son is allergic to chickpeas – who knew. After he refused to eat the first black bean brownies I decided to make chickpea chocolate chip cookies! In theory it was a healthy substitute; however, he took one bite and right away knew he was allergic to them! That was a tough lesson to learn.

However, I persevered and in the end I have found recipes that work for me and my family. When I feed these desserts and snacks to my family and friends, I feel good about it. I know their bodies will be able to absorb and process the nutrients that are in the ingredients. There is the occasion where I have served them store-bought, packaged cookies. I truly feel bad about that. I know that the ingredients used in pre-packaged foods are not top quality and don't fit my criteria for healthy eating. But, sometimes life is busy and I run out of time or energy and I take the easy road. That is life and I try not to worry about it too much. I know that most of the time we make choices that serve our bodies and that is a good thing.

I ask you: what are your favourite desserts or baked goods? Can you take your favourite recipe and change up some of the ingredients to increase the nutritional content? This is what I did and it worked for me. I still enjoy all my favourite baked goods but now I know that my body is benefiting from the ingredients and I never feel deprived, and if I am out somewhere and someone offers me a piece of regular cake, I will usually accept because my journey is not about deprivation or strict dieting. A piece of cake, is not a step backwards, it is simply a piece of cake, I eat it and then I move forward.

Ice Cream

Ice cream is another one of those sweet, delicious treats in life that you shouldn't have to live without. But, most store-bought ice cream is usually high in unhealthy fat, sugar, artificial flavours, and preservatives: all items that I decided were causing problems in my body. So, once again, I asked myself the question: *"How can I make healthy ice cream?"* Sure enough, I started to see posts on Instagram about healthy *#nicecream*. So, I started to experiment with some of the recipes and was shocked at how easy and fun it was to make my own frozen, creamy dessert that is way better than regular, old, store-bought ice cream. If I am going to eat ice cream, I want it to be nutritious and delicious.

The combinations are endless. I have included three of my favourite recipes in the recipe section on pages 222 and 223.

So far in this chapter I have talked a lot about the changes I made to my breakfast, snacks, pizza night, pasta and desserts. I hope that I have given you some ideas on how you can start to make changes to some of your favourite meals or recipes. But, I really need to spend more time talking about vegetables and how I learned to crave vegetables. Yes, you read that correctly, I actually learned to crave vegetables and so, I am dedicating a whole chapter to my new best friend: vegetables.

Chapter 6

Learning to Crave Vegetables

I can tell you with 100% honesty that I now actually crave vegetables. I know what you are thinking: *"Yeah sure! Well that's you – not me! I hate vegetables!"* I hear you; in my past, I was not a huge fan of vegetables either. I struggled to eat two to three servings of fruits and vegetables a day let alone the recommended eight to ten servings. I thought it was impossible and no one walking the face of the planet ate that many servings. It just wasn't realistic. I could easily consume eight to ten servings of simple carbohydrates in a day (in the form of boxed cereals, muffins, bread, pasta and crackers). But, eating eight to ten servings of fruits and vegetables (complex carbohydrates) – forget it! Vegetables were boring and bland and fruit had way too much sugar so I ate very little of these foods! Clearly, I had much to learn and a few things I needed to unlearn.

Again, the road to craving vegetables started with an awareness. I knew I had to get more fruits and vegetables into my body, so I went to work to find new creative ways to incorporate more of these vital foods into my meals. In particular, I needed more vegetables, so I started my journey with soup. Here is my story:

Soup

When I was a kid my favourite soup was canned cream of mushroom with lots of crackers and not too many big mushroom pieces. I could also tolerate tomato soup and if I had to, I could eat chicken noodle soup but only the brand with the small noodles. As a teenager, a friend of mine introduced me to bean with bacon soup: I thought that was good.

Then there was my stepmom's homemade soup. Let me just say that I was not a fan of that soup and I struggled to eat it each time it was served. I don't know who taught her to make that soup. It was probably a recipe passed down from generations ago when ingredients were harder to come by: you wasted nothing and you ate what was put in front of you. I don't know; in any event, I formed an opinion that homemade soup was terrible, and that canned store-bought soup was the only edible soup available.

Occasionally we would go to a restaurant and a bowl of soup was included and served at the beginning of the meal. I never actually ordered soup....who would do that!? However, what I discovered by eating the soup in the restaurants was that soup could actually taste good and even somewhat delicious. But, of course the soup was made by trained chefs who had secret recipes, exotic ingredients and industrial equipment. A person like me would have to stick to canned soups and that is what I did.

It wasn't until 1999 when I was already in my late 30s that I made my first batch of homemade soup. A friend and I had taken a *'Heart-Smart'* cooking course offered through our local continuing education organization. We learned to make several heart healthy dishes including a homemade cauliflower soup. I was amazed at how good it was and how easy it was to make. I made that soup a couple other times and then I went back to buying canned soup.

Eventually my choice of canned soups evolved to the point where I was purchasing soups with chicken and vegetables, beef and barley, lentils and vegetables and occasionally a Tetra Pack of organic, butternut squash soup when it was on sale.

When I finally made the connection that I needed to eat more vegetables and I needed to take my lunch to work, it was these healthier version soups that I turned to. I got into the habit of adding extra vegetables to the canned soups. At first this meant some extra frozen green beans, peas, or corn. Eventually, I started to cook extra vegetables, chicken or beef so that I had leftovers to throw into my soup the next day. These lunches changed so much! They were tasty and filling; they were nutritious and fuelled my body for a busy afternoon.

At some point I remember having a conversation with a friend of mine about canned fruits and vegetables. There was much talk about chemicals leaching from the cans into the food and how toxic these were to our bodies. This was tough for me to hear and absorb but something about this information flipped a switch in my brain and I decided that I needed to figure out a way to make my own soups from scratch.

Then as fate would have it, one day I found myself with a big bag of organic carrots and a head of broccoli that needed to be eaten. I decided to pull out my old cauliflower soup recipe and I applied the same steps to make the carrot broccoli soup: I simply substituted the carrots and broccoli for the cauliflower. The soup turned out great and I was really impressed with myself! If I could make this soup taste good, maybe, just maybe, I could make other soups as well.

Next, I decided to try my hand at butternut squash soup. I found a recipe online and then headed to the grocery store to pick up my first ever butternut squash. I had read somewhere that roasting a butternut squash first was a great way to bring out more flavour so that is what I did. The soup turned out great! Okay, now I was on a roll.

One day I was cleaning out my fridge and I was debating what to do with a big box of mushrooms that were about to expire. Then it hit me – make mushroom soup! So, once again I applied the same principles to make the mushroom soup as I did to make the original cauliflower soup so many years earlier. The mushroom soup was delicious and what was so exciting was that it was homemade! It was delicious homemade soup!

I had discovered that good soup did not have to come from a can or a restaurant. I learned that I too could make a good pot of soup. All I needed was one basic recipe, a few ingredients, average kitchen equipment and a little desire! I was so excited and so grateful for all that I was learning (and unlearning).

Over the last few years, I have expanded my collection of recipes for great tasting soup to include:

- Asparagus and celery
- Leek, potato and broccoli
- Carrot ginger
- Carrot, yam and coconut
- Lentil squash

The list goes on; there is no limit to what you can make.

I often add leftover roasted vegetables, spinach, chunks of cooked chicken or cooked quinoa to my pureed soup. It becomes a complete meal, full of goodness and nutrition. I encourage you to make your own soups as a way to get more vegetables into your body. It is easy, fun, and rewarding.

My basic soup recipe can be found on page 207.

I share my soup story with you not because I think that the way to health and happiness is to learn to make and enjoy homemade soup (although this might be helpful). I am not trying to tell you that if you do what I did then you will be successful on your weight loss journey. You may not even like soup! I share this story because I believe that each and every one of us has eating and cooking experiences that have helped shape and form our belief systems around food. Some of these experiences may be positive and some may not be. I believe that if you want to improve your health and wellness then one of the things that you must do is to look closely at your eating and cooking patterns and pinpoint one or two areas that you can begin to make some healthy, positive changes.

Ask yourself:

- What experiences have you had that have shaped your current belief system?
- Are there things you can change about those belief patterns?
- Is there an experience that you can relive in a more positive way?
- What one thing can you do to give your body more of what it needs or less of what it doesn't?

I grew up believing that good soup came in a can and that homemade soup was awful. My exposure to vegetables as a kid was limited to basic iceberg lettuce salads and overcooked frozen vegetables. I also grew up with very little confidence in myself as a cook.

As I began my wellness journey I identified that I needed to eat less simple carbohydrates and I needed to get more complex carbohydrates in the form of vegetables into my body: soup became my vessel. My soup journey began almost 20 years ago without me really knowing what was unfolding. It started with a class I took where I learned to make cauliflower soup. Fast forward many years and I now make all my own vegetable and chicken stock and I grow many of the vegetables that I use in my soups. I stock my freezer with soup so that at any given time I can go to the freezer, pull out some soup and enjoy the delicious goodness for lunch or dinner.

Learning to make soups using lots of fresh vegetables was one important step that I took on my wellness journey.

Salads

There probably isn't a person alive who has been on a traditional diet who hasn't munched their way through many boring salads. To this day when I hear the word *salad* I have to talk my way through it. Subconsciously I must associate the word *salad* with being on a *diet*....a word that I hate because I spent half my life on a *diet*. To me, salads usually consisted of a plate of iceberg lettuce tossed with a few bits of grated carrots, a couple chunks of cucumber, some diced tomatoes (which I have detested most of my life), and served with a side of celery sticks. Mostly, my salads had no dressing **because I was on a diet**! Ugh!! No wonder I never kept the weight off, who can live on that! Oh the days!

But, I am all grown up now and I have learned a lot. I now know that a salad needs to be more than a plate of food more suited to a bunny rabbit than a human being on the go. A salad needs to satisfy your body's requirement for protein, carbohydrates and healthy fats. It also needs to satisfy your taste bud's desire for an explosion of texture and flavours. It must be colourful and appealing and it absolutely has to taste delicious.

Truthfully, salad making is not my strength. Having said that, I do love a good salad but most of my favourite salad recipes are borrowed from other people who do it better than I do. One of my favourite recipes is for the "*long weekend grilled salad*" from **Oh She Glows**. This salad is delicious and when I eat it my mouth does a happy dance, I feel nourished and fulfilled

Recently, this salad was an inspiration to me when I found myself with some leftover grilled red peppers in my fridge along with some cooked quinoa. I used these ingredients along with a few other items and ended up making the most delicious salad that I have ever made.

Inspiration and motivation can lead to creation. I share my Accidental Quinoa Vegetable Salad recipe on page 210.

My family and I really love Caesar salad and I make it at home often; sometimes I add chunks of chicken and avocado or warm seafood like scallops and prawns, so good! I also enjoy a good spinach salad (with bacon of course). I often order a salad at a restaurant because I know with almost 100% certainty that the salad will taste great and that I will be happy with my choice: I will feel satisfied and my body will be nourished. Restaurant salads always taste great and I like to make notes of the ingredients in the salad so that I can duplicate it at home.

As I continue to learn and grow and expand my knowledge and change my beliefs around the word *salad*, I find more and more delicious salad recipes finding their way into my world. A while ago my life-long friend Shawna and her husband came to visit us. She made a delicious salad that still makes my mouth water when I think of it. I love it when healthy food creates such a reaction in my body.

With Shawna's permission, I have reprinted her sensational spinach salad recipe on page 209.

It really is exciting to learn new things, to challenge our belief systems and to discover that we can do things that we thought only the experts could do! And so, the learning continues.

Learning to crave vegetables has been an ongoing process for me. It hasn't always been easy but, what I have discovered is that when I do eat lots of vegetables my body responds with energy and vitality. My body positively loves it when I feed it lots of vegetables and as a result I continually look for new ways to eat vegetables in as many creative ways as possible. Here are a few other things that I do to get more vegetables into my body.

Roasted Vegetables

Believe it or not, I only learned to make roasted vegetables a few years ago. It is such a simple and easy way to cook vegetables but I honestly never did it before. Then one day a friend of mine was telling me about the roasted vegetables she had made, so I decided to give it a try. I remember calling her to ask her if I could roast celery (because I had celery in my fridge). She said that she had never done it before and so she really didn't know if the celery would roast up good or not. I decided to give it a try. I cut up my potatoes, carrots, cauliflower, onions and celery, tossed them in olive oil, salt and pepper and put them in the oven for about an hour. This was so simple and the vegetables tasted great! The celery, well, it wasn't horrible, but, I never did roast it again.

I now make a big tray of roasted veggies on a regular basis. I include whatever I have on hand: potatoes, yams, carrots, cauliflower, brussel sprouts or butternut squash (I also roast asparagus, peppers, zucchini, green beans and broccoli but find that these don't require as much time to cook so if I am using these vegetables, I add them part way through the cooking process). I cut the veggies up into bite-sized pieces, toss them in olive oil and sprinkle with salt and pepper and sometimes Italian spice mix, garlic or rosemary. I cook them for about 45 minutes in a 375 degree oven, stirring them up once or twice so they brown evenly on all sides.

What is so great about this method of cooking is that the roasting brings out depth in the flavour and I always have lots of leftovers. The following day, I can add the leftover veggies to my scrambled eggs at breakfast, my soup at lunch, and my rice or noodle stir-fry at dinner. Having a big bowl of leftover roasted vegetables makes meal time quick, easy and nutritious and I know that I am getting all the vegetables that my body needs in order to function at its prime.

More Veggies for Breakfast

I have already talked about this but, it is worth repeating: I eat a lot of vegetables at breakfast. I make omelettes loaded with spinach, broccoli, mushrooms and/or asparagus. I scramble eggs with leftover roasted veggies and top with salsa. I make yam waffles and top with spinach, eggs and avocado. I put veggies in my smoothies including, spinach, kale, cucumbers, and precooked beets, yams, carrots and squash. I often steam a big pot of cut-up beets, then lay them out on a cookie sheet and freeze them. Once frozen, I can package them in freezer bags and use them in my smoothies. If I happen to have too much spinach or kale on hand I freeze it too.

One morning I was making myself a smoothie and, among other ingredients, I added frozen spinach, frozen beets and frozen peaches. The resulting "smoothie" was more like ice cream! That turned out to be an accidental, beautiful and delicious morning treat!

I called this creation "Pretty in Pink Frozen Goodness." The recipe is on page 203.

When I start my day with a lot of vegetables, I always feel full longer and I feel nourished and satisfied. I also feel proud and strong because I know that I am fuelling my body for success: I will have more energy for the day. Overall I just feel better when my breakfast includes a good serving of vegetables.

Snacks

Eating raw veggies like cauliflower, broccoli, carrot sticks, cucumber, mushrooms, snap peas, radishes, jicama or celery sticks at snack time is a perfect thing to do, especially when you pair them with a homemade dip. My favourite dips are hummus or tzatziki because I love the flavour and I love the fact that I am adding some protein to my snack. It took me a while but I finally found quick and easy homemade hummus and tzatziki recipes that I really like. I try to stay away from supermarket brands because I prefer better quality ingredients and I much prefer the taste of homemade. There are so many recipes on line. Try a few until you find the one that you like the best. It only takes a few minutes to make your own dips and when you do, you will be much more likely to eat more raw vegetable which will do nothing but benefit your body.

I believe that it is our body's natural state to crave and eat real food, natural food, and nutritious food: food that fuels our cells and makes us feel good. When I start to feel lethargic or tired I only have to look at what I have been eating to answer the question as to why I am feeling the way I am. I am going to summarize my thoughts on eating vegetables by sharing the following with you. I wrote it on October 2, 2015. I have left this unedited because I think these words perfectly sum up how I feel about vegetables.

"I know that I am not eating enough vegetables and I also know that when I do eat lots of vegetables, I just feel better. I don't know exactly what it is that my body needs. Is it the fibre, the nutrients, the slower consumption time (I tend to eat too fast but it's hard to eat a salad fast), or is it the joy of consuming all those colours. I love it when I look at my plate and there are lots of colours on it. It looks happy, I am happy. When my plate looks boring and is lacking in colour I don't think happy thoughts. I think "I need some green" or "where's the colour?" Or "that's kind of bland looking!" I know consciously that I am missing something by the lack of colour on my plate. Physically, I can start to feel the longing for something more. I start to feel unfulfilled, or un-full-filled. In other words: I am not filled with 'stuff' that I need in order to feel fulfilled! (I shudder to think how many countless times I have reached for a donut or bag of cookies when what my body was craving was vegetables!) I can feel it and yet sometimes it takes a while to clue in to what's happening. However, when I do clue in, I can then take action and start the process of eating more vegetables in more creative ways. It doesn't take long. A couple of good servings of vegetables and I am back on track. My body just works better. I feel better in so many ways. For starters, I am more 'regular' thanks to the added fibre. I am less bloated; again, the fibre plays a big role in this. I have more energy, thanks to all the micro and macronutrients that are making their way through my cells giving them the fuel they need to do their job more efficiently. I

sleep better because my body can actually relax more knowing that it isn't deprived of the basic essentials. Overall, I am happier because my body is happier. Eating more vegetables is a great habit to form. Like any other new habit, it may take time to implement and you may forget, or get lazy, or busy, or go through a period where you just feel like pizza instead. I say, don't worry too much about it, but, do get back on the veggie train and take a ride. It really is the best thing for you, and your body will dance with happiness. There is something about the life forces of vegetables that works. I imagine all the living cells of the vegetable plants entering my body and happily and joyfully travelling through my body working at repairing and energizing the cells, tissue, organs and muscles of my body. I have finally learned to listen to my body instead of my taste buds or my mother's voice telling me what to do instead of doing what my body needs to do. I am now wiser and all grown up, so I can listen to my body and feed it what it needs."

If you want to lose weight or get healthier then you are going to have to make changes. You are going to have to find fun ways to move your body and you are going to have to find new and healthier recipes that fuel your body, your mind and your soul. We all enjoy food that tastes good. But, we also need food that is good for you, that is real and that is grown or raised in natural, sustainable ways. Get to know the food you put into your body. Where does it come from? How is it grown? How is it raised? Is it real? Is it life-giving or life-depleting?

Once you start making these changes, you will begin to see and feel the differences and you will be rewarded because each new positive change you make feeds your body, mind and soul in so many ways. There will be no going back because you will have learned new ways that make you feel alive and energetic, and these new, healthy decisions will become a way of life for you.

Your journey is waiting for you to say *"yes!"* Your journey begins when you commit to doing better for your body. The commitment starts with one positive decision, one small change and then it grows one step at a time.

Your journey will unfold differently than mine did. You are unique and beautiful and so too will be the road you travel, but, you are the only one who can take your journey. You hold the key, you make the choices. You get to decide moment by moment how you will live your life.

Choose *healthy* and a whole new world will open up for you. It did for me and I will never go back.

Chapter 7

The More I Learned, the More I Lost

Over the course of my healthy journey I have changed many things about the way I eat. I now consider food as fuel for my body. I have a much better understanding of how food works in the body and although I am far from an expert on the subject I know our bodies need a balanced combination of protein, carbohydrates and healthy fat. I now understand the difference between complex carbohydrates and simple carbohydrates. I came to realize that my body was literally caught in a vicious cycle with all the simple carbohydrates I was eating (cereal, breads, muffins, pasta, bagels, sandwiches, pizza, flour and sugar). The more I ate, the hungrier I was. So, I ate more and continued to gain weight.

Once I finally understood how our bodies process simple carbohydrates, I made the switch. (To repeat: simple carbohydrates turn into sugar in the blood stream, insulin rushes in and converts it into fat for use at a later time.) Armed with this new knowledge, it became pretty easy to start eliminating as many simple carbs as possible and replace them with more complex carbs like fruits and vegetables, healthy fats and more protein.

I learned that fats that come from sources like salmon, nuts, avocados, and olive oil are absolutely essential for the proper metabolism of our food. They protect our cells from damage and they aid in the absorption of vital nutrients. In my past, I avoided avocados and nuts because I knew they were high in fat and calories and I didn't want to get fatter by eating them! This way of thinking is crazy! Your body needs healthy fats. I now know that avoiding these healthy fats in your diet is similar to sending your kids to school and allowing them to learn reading and writing but not allowing them to learn math. It just shouldn't be done; it would be a disaster.

This is pretty much what happens in our bodies too. If we deny our bodies any of the essential nutrients, the result could be disastrous and our bodies could be in danger. We need to pay attention. I now eat these foods often and I love how they work in my body. I often think of these fats as the oils that make my body run smoothly, much like the oil in your car makes it run smoothly. If you remove the oil (healthy fats) your car (body) will cease to function properly.

I learned more about protein as well. I learned that protein is the building block for our muscles, and I am not just talking about body-builder muscles (but of course it builds those muscles too – body-builders love their protein). I am talking about the muscles that each and every one of us needs to carry our bodies throughout the day: muscles that hold our bones together and keep us upright.

I also learned that eating protein with complex carbohydrates is a great way to slow the absorption of the carbohydrates. You may ask, *"But why do I want to slow the process?"* The answer is so that your blood sugar levels stay more consistent, so that you stay satisfied longer, and so that you can absorb the nutrients from the food. High quality protein in the correct amount is essential to the proper function of the body. Sure, your body can exist without adequate protein, but, you are denying yourself and your body if you deprive it of the quality and quantity of protein that it needs.

It took me years to learn about protein and its importance to my body. In my past my main source of protein was meat. In my 20s I worked for several years in the restaurant business where steak and ribs were consistently on my menu. When I moved to the West Coast in my late 20s I was exposed to a lot more fresh fish and chicken and hence I did adapt my eating habits somewhat.

West Coast living also exposed me to a whole culture of people who were living a vegetarian or vegan lifestyle. This did make a lot of sense to me and so, at one point many years ago, I did try living a vegetarian lifestyle for a month by eliminating all forms of meat, fish and chicken. I ate a lot of pasta with various sauces: I ate vegetarian sandwiches, vegetarian pizza, vegetarian soup, muffins, bread, bagels and cream cheese, and some fruit and vegetables. I thought I was doing such a great thing for my body by eliminating all of these animal forms of protein, however, my month of being a vegetarian was a disaster; I gained seven pounds!

Clearly, what I was eating was not working for my body. What I didn't understand at the time was that the lack of protein and increase consumption of simple carbohydrates was most likely causing my weight gain because my body was out of balance and holding on tight to any and all of the food that I was feeding it. What I did know was that by the end of my month I was desperately craving meat, so I made myself a big steak and abruptly ended my experiment at being a vegetarian.

Right now I can hear all of my vegetarian readers say: *"But, there are many non-animal food sources that contain protein."* Yes, I know that now, but, I didn't know that then. What I concluded from my month of being a vegetarian was that it was definitely not for me. But, the problem was that I did not want to go back to eating the amount of meat that I had in the past. So, I made a new goal: I would eat less meat!

In theory this was a great decision; however, what I ended up doing was cutting back on meat (my main source of protein) and increasing my intake of simple carbohydrates (pasta, bread, cereal). As I look back I can clearly see that over the course of most of my life my diet was way out of balance. I was not eating enough protein, but going back to eating large amounts of meat was not an option, so I had no choice but to discover new forms of protein that I had never considered before.

As previously mentioned, one of first things I did was I switched from eating flavoured yogurt to eating **Greek yogurt**. When I looked at the protein and sugar content of several brands of yogurt at my local grocery store, the difference became clear:

- Greek yogurt:
    - Average amount of protein per serving: 16-21grams
    - Average amount of sugar per serving: 3-7 grams
- Flavoured yogurt:
    - Average amount of protein per serving: 3-6 grams
    - Average amount of sugar per serving: 16-21 grams

Unflavoured Greek yogurt became my obvious choice. Admittedly, I pretty much always add fruit to my Greek yogurt or a teaspoon of jam to sweeten it up a bit because it is pretty sour on its own. Nevertheless there is a lot less sugar and a lot more protein in my yogurt than in pre-flavoured and pre-sweetened brands.

The other thing I did to add protein was that I discovered **hemp**

seeds and **flax seeds**. A tablespoon of these little gems adds about 3 grams of protein. I sprinkle them in my smoothies, use them in my muffin recipes, I add them to my scrambled eggs, yogurt and oatmeal. I often use flax seeds in my baking as a replacement for eggs. I simply add:

- 1 tbsp of flax seeds to 2.5 tbsp of water then let the seeds soak up the water for about 5 minutes. What you get is a 'flax egg' which is a great replacement for eggs in vegan baking recipes.

Of course, I don't limit my intake of seeds to hemp seeds and flax seeds; I now regularly eat sunflower seeds, pumpkin seeds, chia seeds, and sesame seeds.

Before I started my healthy journey I never considered **vegetables as a source of protein**. But, as I continued to learn, I discovered that many vegetables contain protein. Common vegetables like broccoli, peas, asparagus, spinach and brussel sprouts are all excellent sources of protein and I eat these often now. I eat them roasted, steamed, or stir-fried. I make soups with them, scramble them in my eggs, put them in smoothies and eat them raw. Including as many of these vegetables as possible into my meals not only adds protein but, these vegetables are also complex carbohydrates and full of goodness for my body.

Another plant-based source of protein that I discovered was **lentils**. Prior to the beginning of my journey I had never cooked lentils before. However, as I started to explore new recipes, I was introduced to a butternut squash and lentil soup from *Oh She Glows*. I have made this recipe many times and I love it. It is delicious, nutritious and full of goodness.

Lentils are also a key ingredient in the base of many vegetarian shepherd pie and 'meat loaf' recipes. Try one of the recipes online and see what you think. Lentils are an excellent substitute for the ground beef traditionally found in these recipes. No one is asking you to give up beef, but, it certainly doesn't hurt to cut back and try some healthy options. This tip worked for me and I hope you find some value in it too.

Other common **legumes** that I became more familiar with are **chickpeas** and **beans**: both of which are high in protein. I now make my own hummus using organic canned chickpeas. I also make curries using chickpeas and I add chickpeas to my salads. There are several recipes online for black bean brownies or cake. I put at least two types of beans in my chili. I love making a simple bean and rice dish that I put in lettuce wraps. Basically I combine cooked rice and black beans with salsa, chopped cilantro and avocado. I then spoon the mixture into lettuce leaves, roll them up and enjoy a quick, delicious, nutritious, wheat-free meal.

Finally, I discovered **quinoa**: probably my most important discovery. What I learned is that quinoa is the only non-animal source of protein that contains all 23 amino acids, making it a complete protein (just like a steak). Quinoa is amazing and has so many uses. I almost always have a container of cooked quinoa in my fridge. I use it to make muffins and quinoa patties. I add it to my soups and scrambled eggs. I mix it with 'cauliflower rice' and Mexican spices to make a filling for tacos. I use it to make stir-fries, pizza crusts and chocolate cake! I love quinoa; it is versatile, nutritious and so easy to make:

-   Simply add 1 cup of quinoa to 2 cups of water, let simmer for 15 minutes (or until water is absorbed), let rest for 5 minutes then serve or refrigerate for use another day.

Funny thing about quinoa is that the first time I made it I served it plain, just like I would serve rice. We didn't like it! So, the bag of quinoa sat in my cupboard for months until I decided I needed to get creative and find ways to use it up. Back to my computer I went, and wow, was I ever surprised to find so many recipes that incorporated quinoa! Now, I can eat pizza and chocolate cake knowing that I am eating protein with each bite; it's a delicious and nutritious thing!

Once I started to eat meals that were much more balanced and virtually wheat-free, my body immediately responded. I ate, and I ate, and I ate, and I started to lose weight. It was truly amazing! I never felt deprived and the hunger pangs that had previously seen me stuffing my face with whatever I could get into it virtually stopped. I felt so much better; I felt sane. I had finally learned how to fuel my body in such a way that I could eat and then get on with my day without experiencing the highs and lows of out-of-control blood sugar levels. I finally felt free from the trap that food had on my body and my mind. This was a major relief and a major contributing factor in my weight loss.

I was retraining myself, I was unlearning old patterns and I was learning and implementing new ones. I exercised, I ate and slowly, very slowly, I noticed that my clothes were starting to feel loose. I would weigh myself and see that I had lost a few pounds. That was exciting.

There were many times however, that I would weigh myself and I would see that I had gained weight. Right now I can hear some people say, *"Why was she weighing herself all the time?"* I know there are many conflicting views about bathroom scales: should we weigh ourselves? How often? Should we just throw the scales out? For me, I have weighed myself my whole life and I have had good days and bad days based around whatever number the scale spat at me. The scale has not always been my friend.

However, this time was different. This time I was not focused on losing weight. This time my focus was on improving my overall health, so my purpose in weighing myself was pure curiosity. My clothes were looser so that must have meant I had lost weight, and usually I had.

After a few months of weighing myself every few days I noticed a real pattern: I would lose two pounds, and then I would gain one. Or I would lose three pounds and then I would gain two. It was up or down every time. When it was up I literally told myself that it would be down next time so I never spend a moment worrying about it. I have learned that the scale can and will change every day because our bodies are constantly changing, constantly processing, absorbing and eliminating the food and drinks we consume. A big glass of water can weigh a pound. So, if I was up a pound I was not worried, it was no big deal.

As the weight continued to come off I remember thinking that there might be something wrong with the scale. First I was down eight pounds, then 12, then 17, then 23, then 27, then 35, then 42! Say what!? The scale must be wrong! But, what about all the people who kept complimenting me: were they wrong too? What about the people who said, *"You are so little!"* *"Who me!?"* It wasn't real. I wasn't on a diet so how could I be losing all this weight?

The truth came when I would pull something out of my wardrobe that I hadn't worn for a long time and it would literally hang off me. I had a little black dress that I pulled out one day to wear to an upcoming event. I probably hadn't worn that dress for about a year. I suspected that I might have to alter the dress, but, there was no way;

that dress was way too big! I knew the dress hadn't gotten bigger so I must have gotten smaller! This was definitive proof that I had indeed lost weight and that the bathroom scale was not broken.

I also remember the second summer of my journey. I had pulled out a pair of shorts that were probably three years old. I had worn them the previous summer and noted that they were looser than in previous years. However, this particular summer when I put the shorts on, they literally fell to the floor! It was unbelievable, but it was true! I had accomplished something I had never in a million years thought I could and what was so amazing to me was that I never once considered myself to be on a diet. I was on a mission to get healthier, to lower my blood pressure, to sleep better, to gain energy, and to take better care of myself. In order to reach my goal I had to make a healthy choice, and then another, and then another. As I fed and moved my body, I started to feel better and look better, and quite naturally the excess weight came off.

Food can be your friend. It can nourish you, give you energy and heal many ailments. But, the wrong food can have the opposite effect. It can leave you wanting and craving more. It can alter your mood. It can suck your energy, leave you restless and create all kinds of havoc in your body.

On my journey I discovered a new way of eating that works for me and makes my body happy. I enjoy knowing that the food I eat most of the time is nourishing, tasty and that it is going to be of positive use in my body. I wonder how many people actually think about the food that they eat.

Do you think about your food?

Do you choose food because it helps the systems of your body move freely to do all the things it needs to do: to digest our food, absorb the nutrients and eliminate the waste?

Is the inside of your body as happy and as cared for as the outside of your body?

Do you bath the inside of your body with nourishing food and drinks the way you bath the outside of your body in cleansing baths, exfoliating rubs and expensive lotions?

The inside of our body is equally as important (if not more important) than the outside of our bodies, yet as a society we spend billions of dollars making the outside of our bodies appealing and pleasant to look at. We buy expensive clothes, get manicures and pedicures, wear makeup, search for the perfect accessories and get our hair done just right. We do all this for the outside of our bodies, but, what do we do for the inside?

What do you do to help the inside be as fabulous as the outside?

Eating healthy food and exercising is not just for the *"health freaks"* or *"privileged few."* What does that mean anyway? Eating healthy nourishing foods and getting more oxygen into your body should be the primary goal of everybody because without your health and vitality the quality and duration of your life could be compromised. It has been said often, that if you don't make time for your health now, then you will have to make time for disease later! The cells of our bodies need to be nourished so that they can protect us from disease. Without proper protection, our bodies will start to break down. I do not want that to happen to you.

So, I challenge you to rethink the role that food plays in your life. You might ask yourself:

- What is the purpose of eating this food?
- Is it to satisfy my taste buds for the whole three seconds while the goodness sits on my tongue?
- Or, is the food going to have benefit to my body for hours to come?

I asked myself these questions a lot and most of the time I could pass on the tempting foods because I knew that the three seconds of pleasure was not worth it. My body deserves more than that. My body desires more than that.

There are times however when my brain is telling me that I am craving something sweet and ridiculous and no matter what I do I cannot talk my brain out of its sugary demands. So, I cave; I eat whatever tempting deliciousness is staring me in the face promising to satisfy my every desire. I devour the gooey goodness like a lion tearing apart a carcass in the Sahara Desert! What could be better, and for a few brief moments, the sweetness comforts me like a warm blanket on a cold day.

The beast has been calmed and I can carry on with my day.

It's true; I do succumb to these indulgences. I don't do it because I am 'treating' myself because to me these indulgences are not a treat. I know these treats are not healthy, I know they are full of sugar and fat and that they contain no nutritional value whatsoever. I also know that they do more harm to my body than good: but, I do it anyway! I do it because I am unprepared or because it's what's available, or because a lifetime of false programming has taught me that it's okay to eat crap and that we deserve these 'treats', just this one time!

When these moments happen (and they do happen and will most likely continue to happen for the rest of my life), first I accept what I have done as a moment of human indulgence and then I move on. I have to say this again; perfection is not the goal, it never was.

Living a healthy, sustainable lifestyle is the goal.

There are going to be greasy fries and hot dogs, birthday cake, chocolate bars, smores, donuts from the drive-thru and take-out pizza with a ridiculous amount of cheese on it. At least in my life there is.

But, these items are the exception not the rule.

80/20 Rule

When I was in sales we had a rule we followed called the 80/20 rule. In general, the rule says that 80% of the sales will come from 20% of the customers. We used this rule as a guideline for prioritizing which customers we spent most of our time and energy on. In theory, we were supposed to spend most of our time with those 20% of customers who gave us 80% of our sales.

In my wellness journey I have come across the 80/20 rule again. I have heard it stated many times that:

A successful weight loss can be contributed
80% to the foods we eat and 20% to the exercise we do.

In other words, what we eat has way more impact on our weight loss than how much we exercise. Think about it: we eat at least three meals a day, but we are lucky if we exercise three times a week. The quality and quantity of food that you consume will have a far bigger impact on your weight loss journey than how many miles you run, how many steps you take, how many sit-ups you can do, or how much weight you can lift.

Even during my marathon training, I found that even though I was burning over 3000+ calories a week during my runs, I actually gained weight during my training. Some people will say that it was because I was building strong leg muscles, which is partially true, but the truth is that I was still learning to eat the proper quality and quantity of food that my body needed in order to sustain me before, during and after those long runs.

Don't kid yourself into thinking that you can exercise your way into a new, healthier version of yourself without changing your diet. In the past I tried to exercise my way to a thinner version of myself and had moderate short-term success. However, the demands I placed on my body without proper nutrition only backfired on me and I eventually stopped exercising and gained back my weight and then some!

Proper nutrition and exercise are teammates and they will work wonders in your body if given the chance. I stand firm in my belief that you need a balance of proper nutrition and exercise in order to successfully lose weight and keep it off.

Taking the 80/20 rule one step further, let's talk more about our food choices. There is much written about the success people have had by eating healthy, balanced meals 80% of the time. I have a friend, Patti Fleury, who was diagnosed with Crohn's disease more than 20 years ago. After many years of suffering she went to a naturopathic doctor who suggested that she eliminate wheat, dairy and sugar from her diet. He suggested that if she could eat this way 80% of the time then it would significantly reduce the pain and inflammation she was suffering from. Naturally, my friend followed her doctor's advice and sure enough her symptoms were greatly reduced. She went on to write a book about her experience called *Life After Crohn's: 5 Steps to Total Wellness*. In her book, she documents how changing her diet (and sticking to the plan 70-80% of the time), has transformed her life from one of constant pain and suffering to one of joy and vitality. I would highly recommend reading this book: it is a fascinating account about the power of food in the body.

Some diets allow for a *cheat day* where the participants are allowed to eat whatever they want one day per week. Taking this concept one step further, someone has actually designed a diet called *"The 80/20*

Diet". I don't follow this diet plan (or any other one,) but the concept makes sense to me.

Without planning it, I would say on average this is how I choose to live: around 80% of the time I eat high quality, nutritious, organic, colourful food that provides life-giving energy and fuels my body for success. The other 20% of the time I eat what is put in front of me, or what my mind is telling me that I can't live without, or what is readily available. This way I am not in a daily battle to live up to unrealistic expectation, follow ridged plans, and I don't have to deal with feelings of failure. This has worked well for me: it is stress and guilt-free and that's a good thing.

Having said that, I don't justify eating a cream-filled donut covered in chocolate because I had oatmeal for breakfast and a salad for lunch. I don't plan the 20% of my less-than-healthy indulgences. I actually strive to eat healthy 100% of the time because eating healthy, whole food makes me feel better and that is my main goal. However, I know that 100% is not realistic for my lifestyle, because sometimes the fridge isn't stocked and there are no healthy snacks prepared, and sometimes I am tired and need something quick and easy and 'tasty', then I choose foods that fall into the 20% category because that's life.

If you can aim to eat healthy foods 80% of the time your body will be so happy and so satisfied and when you do face indulgences you can't resist, you will have the confidence, the knowledge and the power to know that this indulgence will not set you back, that it is not cheating and it will not throw you off your plan. You will know that this indulgence is part of the plan: it is within the 20% of your food choices that don't have to be perfectly healthy, and that is also a good thing.

Eating healthy, real, whole foods 80% of the time is an attainable goal, it is realistic, it is doable and it allows room for pizza night, birthday cake, ice cream and gooey donuts.

On a final note about the 80/20 rule: please don't get hung up on the numbers and don't make the mistake of counting how many bites of *healthy* you ate vs. how many bites of *unhealthy*. Strive to eat as many healthy meals as you can, but, leave room for life's little indulgences, leave room for celebration, leave room for trips down memory lane. Listen to your body; make choices that will nourish your body, your mind and your soul. Your health depends on it.

Once again, if you are struggling with your weight, if you aren't feeling good, if you have aliments, if you want to look and feel healthier then you are going to have to make changes to what you eat and drink and you are going to have to move your body. There is no pill, there is no secret recipe, there is no magical formula, there is no 'how to' guide, there isn't going to be a personal chef and fitness coach who show up at your door to do it for you. This is your gig! This is your job. It's up to you to take control of the reigns of your life and steer your choices in a new direction. You have the power, you have the ability.

Ask more of the food you put into your body. Say *"yes"* to foods that nourish and energize you and learn to say *"no"* to foods that serve no purpose other than a few seconds of false bliss. Start to move your body more. There are no excuses! Your body is naturally designed to move. Be good to your body, it really does deserve the best you can give it.

Chapter 8

Facing the Truth and Saying Goodbye

Sometimes in life we have to say goodbye to things that no longer serve us. This might mean saying goodbye to a job, a relationship, the town you live in, the foods you eat or the habits you have formed.

Change for most people is not easy. We are creatures of habit and will often continue to do the same thing over and over and over again even though we know it is not a healthy choice and we long for something different. The habits we form are hard to change because our brains get stuck. Most of us are guilty of spending most of our lives content within our self-imposed comfort zone; even if the comfort zone is less than desirable. Generally people fear the unknown and resist change.

But, in order to grow or to change we have to step outside of our comfort zone. We have to do some things differently. We have to tread in waters that we have never experienced before. This is how we learn, this is how we change, and this is how we grow. On my wellness journey I made changes very, very slowly, one thing at a time, one decision at a time.

As I learned and gained knowledge I knew I had to let go of some old ways of thinking to make room for new, healthy patterns. I wanted to make the changes; I was ready for something better, something healthier, and something positive. Saying goodbye is seldom easy but, I found a fun way to say goodbye to some of my unhealthy habits.

Saying Goodbye to Bread

One night I was inspired to write a goodbye letter to bread, much like you might write a letter to end an unhealthy relationship. In my case, I wasn't breaking up with a boyfriend; I was breaking up with bread. (Actually, I was breaking up with wheat, but bread was my target in this letter.) I hope you enjoy the humour in this letter:

Dear Bread,

You have been my friend for a long time. You were there for me morning, noon and night. You were a constant companion and I relied on you more than I should have. But, as I step away from you now, I realize that you were not good for me. I did not realize until after I left you that you made me feel bad; I felt bloated and puffy and although the taste and texture of you in my mouth was a good thing, that's where the goodness ended. Once you were in my belly things got ugly and uncomfortable. It took me years to realize that perhaps there was a better way; perhaps I could find foods that were delicious and satisfying not only for my taste buds, but also for my insides too. Fair is fair. I now see that there is no point causing pain and discomfort to one area of my body just so another area can relish in selfishness. It's just not worth it anymore!

So, I am sorry to say that it is time to say goodbye to you as I know you. I must replace you with other healthier, well-rounded, more nurturing food items. I now see that hanging out with you leads to so many other problems. In short, you are not good for me. So, adios dear bread: farewell, goodbye!

In health,

Rhonda

Chapter 8

What Lies Beneath the Cake?

Saying goodbye to traditional cake, donuts and cookies made with wheat and sugar and unhealthy fat was also a positive choice that I had to make. Here I share my thoughts on these sweet indulgences that I wrote one night after turning away from cake:

Last night after our run, our run club was giving out pieces of cake to celebrate someone's birthday. I started to walk towards the cake and then realized that I really, truly did not want a piece of cake. I wanted to enjoy the blissful feelings of just finishing a great run. My lungs were doing a happy dance, my muscles were vibrating with excitement and the smile on my face did not need cake to smear it away. Now, don't get me wrong, cake can be a good thing and cake should be part of life. But, on my terms, not because it's sitting there trying to be tantalizing and sending out false promises of joy and bliss.... Sorry cake! Not this time! This time, I walk away, and the moment I turn around I feel a great big 'YES' run through my veins and I feel the happy dance all over again! This, my friends, is what control is all about. It's not about deprivation, it's not about going without. It's about making the decision that's best for the higher good. At that particular moment in time, the best decision was to turn around and walk away! Try it next time there is a temptation facing you spewing out promises of joy and happiness, comfort and joy. But, "I deserve it," I can hear you say. What do you deserve? Why do you think that cake is a reward? It's not a reward! It's a trick, it's a test, it's a temptation and that is it. It's most likely not even that good. It promises stuff it can't deliver for anything more than a brief moment in time that it sits on your tongue and then the promise is gone! So fast, and somehow we buy into that promise over and over and over again. Next time look that piece of cake in the face

113

and ask it to be honest with you about its promises. Challenge it. Don't just let it win you over with its false promises so quickly. Ask questions and really take a minute to ask yourself if you believe this piece of cake. Maybe walk away and decide to think about it for a minute. There may be times that the piece of cake yells back at you **"Wait, come back, you and I aren't finished, I have more promises to tell you. I promise to make you feel good. I promise I will be the best thing you ever tasted. I promise that I won't just sit on your hips. I promise to nourish your body and give you lots of energy!!"** *Lies…all lies!!!*

But what happens when you do turn back towards the cake? (And I am sorry to say, but, you most likely will turn around and head back to the cake table from time to time, and that's called life.) The thrill of the promises catches you off guard and there you stand with the cake at your lips and there is magic in the air. I know; I have been there time and time again. The sweet, creamy, deliciousness is overwhelmingly satisfying, even for the brief few seconds. The next thing that happens the second that you swallow: the pleasure of the sweetness slowly starts to fade and the ugly cousin called 'guilt' starts to rise from the depths of your soul and starts to cloud your veins like a dark storm rolling in from the distance. Here it comes, and there is nothing you can do about it. The storm is eminent. There is little you can do but buckle down and ride its nasty wave. The regret and the sadness take over and you sit there for hours feeling bad! Wow! When are we going to get it? When are we going to realize that no tantalizing, heavenly sweet, creamy, delicious treat will ever deliver the things it promises?

We need to learn to recognize the pattern. We need to come up with a plan of action for the next time the temptation is staring us in the face and drawing us closer with false promises. We need to change our way of thinking and learn to ask questions about each and every thing we consume. We need to learn to say, "no, I don't think so", "not this time", or "I don't believe you" when faced with a decision to believe the lies or not. We need to learn to look at the choices we have. We need to plant our feet on the ground and put our own personal well-being in the forefront. What is best for you? Will the food you are staring at nourish you? Where is the real pleasure: in the cake or in the triumph of passing up on the cake? My friends, I am here to tell you that there isn't even a comparison. The joy you seek, the pleasure, the comfort, the deliciousness you crave, is not in the cake. It hides in the ability to say "no" to those imposters. Saying "no" and taking back your power is beyond anything that any piece of cake will ever have the ability to provide!

The Dreaded Bathroom Scale

Like most people who have spent most of their life on one diet or another, losing and regaining weight, I have always kept in close touch with my bathroom scale. It has been my friend and my enemy. It has dictated over and over if I am going to have a good day or a bad day. I know people who don't even have a bathroom scale; this, I still don't understand! However, as I continue on my wellness journey, I have learned to give away less of my power to my bathroom scale. I learned that a pound or two or three one way or the other doesn't warrant the emotions that go along with the number. In the past if I lost a couple of pounds I was elated (and usually celebrated with cake!!). If the scale showed me a number that was higher than I had hoped, I would immediately start feeling bad about myself and most likely I would grab a chocolate bar or two and sit in the corner for hours licking my wounds. How ridiculous!!

I have learned that the scale will go up and the scale will go down and that's it: my journey stays the same. Having said that, there are times when I know I have gained a few pounds because I have gotten lazy and my healthy eating habits have slipped. That's life; I carry on. I know how to turn things around – I make a positive, healthy choice. I wrote the following one day when I knew I was up a few pounds but refused to play the same old game where I stepped on the scale and it made me feel bad. Instead I made a choice to say "no" to the scale. I hope you enjoy the humour in it.

Dear Bathroom Scale,

I can hear you calling my name, but, I am choosing to ignore you. You see, I know what you will do if I step on you: you will spit out some ridiculous number at me that will just make me feel bad about myself and I don't want to feel bad. I want to feel good, so I am sorry but I will have to pass up on your offer to make me feel bad. Now, don't get me wrong, I know that you have been there for me many, many times and you have brought a great big smile to my face on countless occasions. You have supported me on my journey and even continued to be there like a faithful companion even when I jumped up and down on you! You were even there encouraging me and supporting me after I had chosen to hide you away in the closet for a while. But, alas, I now see you for who you truly are. I was addicted to your positive feedback, when it happened. But, you don't always give me the positive feedback I desire. Sometimes you tell the ugly truth or at least the truth as you see it. You wrap my success or failure up in a number and I now know there is so much more to it than that. The 'truth' you tell is only a small part of my story and not the best part. So, for that reason, I am going to stay away from you for the next several days, maybe even weeks. I don't need you to tell me that I have gained weight (aka – that I have made some bad choices which have resulted in a temporary storage of excessive consumption, or in other words – I have ate way too much of the wrong things and/or not enough of the right things). I know that I have gained weight, but, I also know that I know what to do about it. The most important thing that I need to do is to feel good about myself and make positive changes going forward. You see, I know from repeated experience that if I step on you and you show me a number that I don't like, then I will feel bad. My mind will tell me nasty things that aren't true and frankly I don't want to hear those things anymore. So, thank you for trying to coax me onto you but, I am going to pass this time. This time I choose to stay positive, this time I choose to focus on the progress I have made and the things I have learned so far on my journey. I will not allow you to make me feel bad. You are not my enemy, you are a friend, but one that I have to set boundaries with and boundaries are good for both of us. You are welcome to stay in my life, but on my terms, not yours! Thank you my friend.

Your partner in healthy, happy weight,

Rhonda

The Love of My Life: Potato Chips, Oh How I Love Thee!

For me, love equals potato chips; plain, salty, crunchy, addictive potato chips. I love them and it is an unhealthy love affair and I know it. Even after I lost my excess weight I still ate bag after bag of potato chips. Then sometimes after I finished my bag of potato chips I would dig into my husband's bag of potato chips. I love the word 'potato chips': it has such a nice sound to it. It makes me happy; however, I also know that all those potato chips are not good for me.

At one point I decided I needed portion control so I bought individual bags of potato chips. It wasn't long before I realized that one bag of potato chips was not a full portion. I needed more, so I had another small bag and then another. So much for portion control! In a nut shell, I was addicted to potato chips and ate them almost every day and I ate them like a vulture, all along knowing that eating all these chips was not a healthy choice. Additionally, I know that devouring bag after bag of chips was counterproductive to the message I was trying to spread about living a healthy lifestyle and fuelling my body for success. I felt like a fraud!

Learning to say "no" to potato chips has been my most difficult challenge: one that I am still working on. I have since decided that I am not a fraud, I am a real person with an obstacle to overcome and as I continue to learn and grow and make healthier choices, I have had to confront my addiction to those nasty, delicious, crunchy, salty chips .

A while back, my son and I were watching a documentary on TV about the destruction of the rain forests in South America to make room for planting trees for the purpose of producing more palm oil which is used by fast food companies and potato chip manufacturers!! That made me sick to my stomach! How devastating, and here I was contributing to the problem day after day after day!! How sickening! That bit of news helped a switch go off in my brain. For a long time, I didn't eat my favourite brand of chips and I felt great about that.

However, as life happens, those nasty bags of chips have found their way back into my grocery cart on several occasions. I need to constantly remind myself of the devastation to the rain forests and my goal to live a healthy lifestyle; then I can make wiser choices. I have found some brands of chips that are healthier and sustainable and I do enjoy those very much. There are brands that use other root vegetables like parsnips, beets, sweet potatoes, yams and non-gmo, stone-ground corn, along with quinoa, flax seeds and sesame seeds. They also use more sustainable and healthier oils in their manufacturing process. The best brands are found in the health food section of your supermarket.

Read the labels: look for **non-gmo, sustainable, organic**. When I eat these chips I feel better about my choices and time and time again I find that the healthier chips are much more satisfying and not so crazily addictive. I can often enjoy a bowl full and then I am satisfied.

Yes, they are still chips, but I can munch away knowing that I am not destroying the rain forest and I am not polluting my body with unhealthy fats and who knows what else. This is a step in the right direction. So, I take the wins and celebrate my progress because my wellness journey is exactly that: it is a journey. I am not there yet but each day I carry on because health, happiness, longevity and vitality are my reasons for the choices I make and the lifestyle I choose to live.

I encourage you to think about unhealthy foods or habits that you need to say goodbye to. Don't worry about trying to say goodbye to every bad habit at once. That plan is not realistic and will set you up for failure. Pick one food item or one habit and make a plan to change or eliminate the habit.

Maybe write your own letter to the food or habit that you need to change. Look it in the face and tell it exactly how you feel. Don't hold back. Tell it the good things and the bad. Then tell it what you want. Tell it that you want better, you deserve better, and your body needs better. Be loving and kind but give that bad habit a kick to the curb. You don't need it anymore.

Maybe you can't eliminate the food or behaviour completely. Maybe you need to set new, healthy boundaries around the food or habit. Maybe you need to swap it out for a healthier option. Do what needs to be done. I was successful at greatly reducing the amount of bread I eat; I swapped out traditional cake for cake made with healthier ingredients. I took back the control that the bathroom scale had over my life and I am choosing healthier chips these days.

Practice saying **"no"** to tempting indulgences; take back control over foods or habits that are currently holding you hostage. I had to weed through the lies that certain foods told me and as I changed my ways I started to peel away the layers of fat that were holding me back.

I practiced and I practiced. I am not perfect, I still sabotage myself some days. But, I have learned so much and changed so many of my old ways, so much so that I can never go back to the way I was. I have travelled down a new road and it's beautiful and it feels good. It feels right. It feels like home. Learn to say goodbye to foods or habits that no longer serve the healthier version of you that is emerging. Once you do, there will be no going back.

Chapter 9

Exercise

I struggled to write this chapter on exercise for several months. I was paralyzed by the thought: *"what can I possibly say about exercise that hasn't already been said."* I also know that I am far from an expert on the subject. There are so many highly qualified people who can tell you all the benefits that exercise has. These experts and exercise enthusiasts will all tell you the same thing: exercise is good for you. It will tone your muscles which will help you lose weight, which will make you look better, which will make you feel better, then you will sleep better, your stress will be reduced, you will live longer and stronger, you will be calmer, happier and healthier if you exercise! Blah, blah, blah......! We have heard it all before and we all know that exercise is good for us.

So, what can I say to make a difference? What can I say that is unique and profound? What words will make that little switch in your brain go off? You know that switch where you have an aha moment and you will proclaim, *"OMG, I never thought of it that way before!"* And when that switch goes off I want to know that you will run to your closet and dig through your stuff looking for the running shoes you bought two years ago. Then you will find some shorts and a t-shirt and finally, you will head out your front door and go for a walk! Hallelujah! That's what I want to motivate you to do: I want my words to be the fuel and the inspiration you need to move your body. But, what are those words? I don't know, but I am going to give it my best shot:

- Exercising and being fit is awesome! (No, too simple and vague.)
- Exercising is like the best massage you ever had in a tropical country on the beach, but it's a massage on the inside of your body! (How's that? Do you feel what I mean?)
- Exercise is like putting crispy, cool cucumbers on your tired eyes and breathing in the freshness and naturalness of it all. But the air and the crispness refresh the inside of your body.
- Exercise is to your body what an ice cold glass of lemonade is to your mouth on a hot summer day.
- Exercise is refreshing, it's nourishing, it's invigorating, it's life-giving, it's energizing, and it's as important for the well-being of your body as water, food, sunshine and love.

Yet, if exercise is all these things why do so many people ignore this important and vital link in their health? I believe that some of the answers could be because it's hard, it hurts sometimes, it's boring, maybe it's too expensive, or maybe it's too time consuming. There is a part of me that wants to say, *"blah, blah, blah again….excuses, excuses!!"* But, I am too nice for that. Instead I will say that I agree. I agree that it can be hard and it can hurt. I also agree that it can be boring and expensive and it can be time consuming.

But, I also know the other side of fitness. I know the feeling of pure exhaustion and exhilaration. I know the power behind the pain and the joy in accomplishing a fitness goal. So how do you build a bridge from painful and boring to power and joy? Well my friends, it comes about much the same way as changing what you eat; you take it one step at a time, one choice at a time.

"But, what is the first step?" you might ask. I am going to offer up as an answer:

"Get Rid of Your Excuses"

Your excuses will hold you prisoner for your entire life if you let them. Excuses are lies we use to protect ourselves from failure, pain or embarrassment. Excuses are misleading information we use to explain why we have chosen not to exercise. Excuses need to be put in their place. Let's look at some of the top excuses people often use to explain why they don't exercise.

"It's Hard!"

True: It can be hard, but the good news is that each and every time you get out and exercise you will get a little bit stronger and then a little bit stronger after that. When you want to use the excuse that it's hard just remember that anything you are not used to doing is hard the first time you do it. Learning to walk was hard. You most likely fell down many times before you mastered the fine art of walking. Learning to tie your shoes was hard. Raising children is hard. Starting a new job is hard. Writing this chapter was hard. Most things worth pursuing were initially hard at the beginning, but the rewards, the payoff, is worth the effort put forth, over and over again.

If you have been sedentary for a while it will be hard for you to start an exercise program, it will be hard to show up and it will most likely be hard to keep up with the others that have been doing the exercise for a while. But, the amazing thing is that your body and your mind will adjust to what you give it. If you find it hard to climb a set of stairs but decide to push yourself to climb the stairs over and over again, your body will adjust and soon you will see improvements in your strength and stamina. Soon you will be able to climb the stairs a number of times before reaching the point of exhaustion. Yes, at first it will be hard, but the more you persist, the easier it will get. Soon your body will look at those stairs and think, *Easy peazy – let's go!"*

The hardest thing about starting an exercise program is getting started. But, start you must if you want to experience the joy of physical fitness. Just do it one step at a time and before you know it you will arrive at a beautiful place and you will not want to go back where you came from. I promise!

"It Hurts!"

I will agree that exercising can hurt. It can hurt if you push yourself too hard and cause too much damage to your muscles. It can hurt if you get hit by a high speed ball flying through the air. If can hurt if you trip and fall and skin both hands, both elbows and both knees. I know because I have experienced all these pains. Thankfully, I have never broken a bone while exercising or participating in a sport, but many people have. Yes, it's true; you can get hurt if you exercise. Having said that, I would never trade my fitness level for a safe seat at the side of the game, never!

The benefits of physical fitness far outweigh any pain that I have experienced. Plus, the good news is that getting physically fit does not have to hurt. A proper exercise routine should start out slow and gradual. Ease your way into your chosen exercise. Start low and slow and build up gradually. Your body will respond beautifully if you treat it with love and respect and give it time to adjust. Your body wants to exercise. It wants to move. It will welcome the change but you have to be gentle and nudge it along slowly with kindness and patience.

Don't hit the gym and do 10 rounds of a weight you can barely lift. Don't put on your running shoes and run 5km the first time out. Don't go to an advanced bootcamp class and expect to keep up. Be gentle and be kind to your body and it will reward you with increased energy, improved posture, and renewed self-confidence. You will sleep better, you will look better, you will feel better, and you will think clearer and you will be happier.

There is much written about *"no pain, no gain," "go big or go home,"* and *"do or die."* If those are words that motivate you, then by all means go for it. Listen to your body. What words nudge you forward? For me, I don't believe in pushing myself until it hurts. Now don't get me wrong, I do push myself, but, I stop before the pain sets in. I have had to learn this the hard way. To be perfectly honest, I am not sure I won't ever push myself too hard again. But, I am much better at listening to my body these days and rarely exercise to excess. Truthfully, I am a bit of a wimp; I don't like pain.

For several years now I have had issues with my neck and shoulders. They are a weak spot for me. Again and again I have tried to strengthen them by doing what I thought I should be doing: neck, shoulder and arm exercises. But, each and every time, I have ended up with such neck and shoulder pain resulting in headaches, lack of sleep, lack of concentration and an inability to perform my other exercises. I finally have learned to be gentle and kind while exercising my neck, arms and shoulders. When they start "talking" to me, I stop and listen. I slowly and gently work my upper body. I don't push it, and I am much further ahead because of it! I will never win a weight lifting competition because I use the lightest weights and I am okay with that. For me: less pain equals gain.

I believe that exercising shouldn't hurt. I believe that exercising is meant to heal and strengthen. I also believe that it is meant to stretch your body so that you are pushing your boundaries. But, that's the key: push your boundaries, not someone else's! We are all unique and amazing: we all have different strengths and weaknesses, different levels of tolerances, different pain thresholds. Listen to your body! What is it telling you? If you pay attention, it will tell you when enough is enough. Sometimes, less is more!

"It's Boring!"

Yes, I agree, exercising can be boring, but from my experience the boredom is often an indication that I am not doing the best exercise for me, or that it's time to switch things up. Often the thing that needs to be switched up is my attitude, and the thing that flips the switch on my attitude is to exercise.

Boredom in exercise is a pretty common thing. For me, lifting weights at a public gym is beyond boring. I prefer a faster paced activity and I prefer to be outside exercising. But, I only learned this after buying a gym membership, trying the weight routine and finding myself hating it – it was too boring for me. On the other hand, there are so many people who love the hustle and bustle of the weight room at the gym. I am not one of those people.

Many years ago I attended aerobics classes on a fairly regular basis. However, I found myself getting bored with it after about two years. The music was the same, the steps were the same – I got bored.

I also have a notion that running alone is boring – it's something I dread. I much prefer running with a group or a buddy. It's great to have someone to talk to along the route and the time seems to go by quite quickly. There are times however that due to busy schedules I find it necessary to run by myself. I usually start the run by dreading the boredom. However, a funny thing happens on the road: the boredom starts to leave and the joy of running starts to fill the gap. Where I once felt dread, I now feel joy and life. I love it when my body proves my mind wrong. My mind may be trying to talk my body out of running, but my body is now strong and determined and it loves a good run.

If you find yourself bored, you need to change the exercise, change the location, change the experience, find a new workout buddy or go buy yourself some fun new workout gear: that will put pep in your step. Our minds and our bodies love variety so don't get stuck in boredom; get creative and do something different. Your body and your mind will love it!

"It's Too Expensive!"

There is no question about it; exercising and fitness can be expensive. Depending on your sport of choice you can literally spend thousands of dollars getting your body in shape and enjoying the fun and thrill of so many exhilarating sports. You can spend your money on memberships, equipment, footwear, clothing, personal trainers, coaches, travel, entrance fees, physiotherapy, massage, and nutritional products all meant to support you on your journey. I can say with all honesty that my fitness journey has cost me a fair amount of money. But, I can also say that every dime has been worth it. In life we spend our money and our time on things that make us happy and on things that we value. For me, I value physical fitness over designer clothes or handbags. I value health and vitality over an expensive restaurant meal. My expendable income is limited, so I choose wisely: I choose physical fitness.

I have heard many people say that they can't afford to join a club, or they can't afford the equipment, or they can't afford the membership. I believe that what they are really saying is that they don't see the value in spending their hard earned money on a particular item or sport or physical fitness activity. Sometimes it takes a special circumstance or a lucky break to show us that we can actually afford what it is that our heart desires.

Years ago I started to gain an interest in yoga. There was a new yoga studio opening up in town and I was fortunate to have purchased a one month pass for at least half its value at my son's annual school fair. I really enjoyed the yoga classes that I attended that following month but decided I couldn't afford to buy a monthly pass. I did choose however to buy a 10-class pass which I spread out over two or three months. Attending these classes was a special treat for me but honestly I never gained the benefit of yoga because my attendance was so spread out; there was no connection with the practice. After my 10-class pass was used up I only ever purchased promotional short-term memberships that I thought I could afford. I only ever really dabbled in yoga, but always hoped to grow my practice somehow, someway, someday.

As fate would have it, one night I attended a local wine and art walk in our downtown core. Although I was very late to the gathering I did make it to the final three or four businesses. One of the businesses was another new yoga studio that was scheduled to open within a month or so of the art and wine event. The final business was a financial institute where everyone could enter their name in a draw for the grand prize basket worth over $1000. It was full of gifts from all the local businesses that were participating in the event. Within the basket was a three-month unlimited membership to the new yoga studio. Guess who won the basket? I did! The basket was amazing, full of so many wonderful items but the thing that I was most excited about was the three-month unlimited membership to the new yoga studio!

Those three months of free yoga was a huge gift to me. Not only did I attend regularly, but, I also had the freedom to try lots of different types of yoga. I tried out different teachers and really embraced and used the gift for all its worth. But, the most important thing that I gained from the gift was the knowledge and the reassurance that I can afford yoga. It has become as important in my life as running, eating and sleeping. Sure, I have gone for periods of time when my membership has expired and I get busy and don't make it to a yoga class for a month or so. I don't get stuck and dwell on it. I know that yoga is important and when the time is right, I get my butt back to my mat and all is good. My body, my mind and my soul all benefit from yoga and it is something I will practice until the day I die. It is important! It is of great value to me. Yes, it costs money – but, it's worth every dime and then some!

Please don't use the excuse that exercising is too expensive, because that's not the truth! For one, there are so many things you can do that cost nothing. Take walking for instance: it's free and so easy to do. There is no excuse. If you can afford a good pair of running shoes, go for a run. There are free run clubs around that not only welcome newcomers but encourage them to join. Take up hiking; such a great sport. Play tennis, you just need a racket and a couple of tennis balls. You can rent exercise videos at the library or watch and participate in countless workout routines on YouTube. People often sell used fitness equipment for a fraction of what they paid for it. And sometimes they even leave equipment at the side of the road for free.

Never let the almighty dollar stand between you and your fitness goals. If you want to get fit there are countless ways you can go about it, and you will be supported. But, you need to decide for yourself what it is you want to do, and then you need to go do it!

"It's Too Time Consuming!"

"I don't have time to exercise," you say.
I say: "You don't have time not to!"

A very powerful thought came to me a while back and I believe it to be true to my core:

A magical thing happens when you make time to exercise:
You will automatically have time for other things!

Us runners know this well. When we are tired, overwhelmed, with lists of things to do, what do we do? We go for a run! Sounds crazy right? The thing is that running helps clear our minds, and helps us focus on our other priorities. After a run, our bodies and our minds are refreshed and we are better able to tackle the rest of the day and get done what needs to be done. There were times when I was training for my marathon that I would be out with the group for four to five hours. I would then return home, do my chores around the house, spend time with my family and still have energy to make a proper dinner. Oh sure, maybe I should have vacuumed instead, maybe I should have worked in the garden more or finished painting the hall. The thing is, all those things can wait because I believe my health and well-being is the most important thing in my life, because without my health I have nothing.

My fitness and health allow me to do things that others only dream of. My health and fitness add quality to my life. I am more alive, more joyful, more adventurous, more present, more grateful, more confident and calmer when I am physically fit. A sparkly clean house lasts for about 30 seconds. A good workout lasts for hours, even days. A good healthy, strong body will add years to your life. It's about priorities, and for me, my health is my priority.

You say, *"But, exercise is not my priority, my kids and my husband and my job are my priority."* Well, how about this: isn't taking care of yourself a priority so that you can better take care of your family and other responsibilities? You know the drill: *"put on your own oxygen mask first before assisting others."* I love that and I think about it often. I never feel guilty about making time for myself. I am a much happier, well rounded person when I do. When I am happier I have more to give to my family which makes them happier. It's a win-win situation. I want the best for my family and taking care of me is an important thing I can do. So, I fit in my workout wherever I can. Sometimes I get my workout or run done early in the morning. Sometimes I exercise mid-day. And there are lots of fitness classes or running groups in the evening. I know the benefits and I know how good I will feel after a workout so I do what needs to be done. I will never apologize for the time or the money I spend taking care of myself.

Don't rob yourself of the experience of fitness and don't use the excuse of not enough time. We all have the same 24 hours in a day. Sure, some people work more hours or have longer commutes, or have more kids demanding their time. Life is busy for everyone. If you have a really busy family life then incorporate fitness into your family time; go for a hike together, toss a ball, play Frisbee, ride bikes together. Or, if your kids already play sports or dance two to three nights a week then use this time to get some exercise yourself. Or, get up early and get your workout done before the kids are even out of bed. I know that most of the women in the 6:00 am bootcamp class are rushing off to work right after class or they are rushing home to get kids up and off to school. But, they have all made a commitment to themselves and they are leading healthy, active lifestyles and are excellent role models for their children. Don't use your kids or your family as an excuse not to exercise, use them as your inspiration and motivation why you must exercise.

If you work full time during the day you might choose to exercise on your lunch hour. My sister Allona has exercised on her lunch hour for years. She would far sooner go for a 45 minute run on her lunch hour than to sit on her butt in the lunch room trading weekend plans with the other staff. There are other times for socializing with your coworkers. Lunch time is my sister's time and I admire her dedication to herself. Again, it's about priorities and forming new habits, and then turning those habits into a way of life. Once you start to exercise and to feel the benefits you will know. And once you know the feeling, you will want to experience it again and again.

There is no excuse for any able-bodied person not to exercise. So put down your excuses and put on your shoes. Our bodies are designed to move and to be strong and active and self-healing. Do your body a favour; go for a walk, take a class, hike, swim, bike, dance, jump, stretch or strengthen. It doesn't matter what you do, but just do something. You and you alone are the one who holds the key to the "start" button. So, push the button, start the process and enjoy the ride to physical aliveness. You won't ever regret it!

Why You Must Exercise

Once again I struggle with how to start this part of the chapter. I barely passed biology all those years ago and really, I can get through my life without having to know all the complicated yet fascinating things that happen to our bodies as we age, as we exercise, or as we sleep. There are plenty of books written to explain the physiology behind exercise and the human body so I am going to leave that to the experts.

What I will share is that I do know that our bodies are designed to move and move they must. Our bodies rely on us to get the oxygen flowing. Sure, we do get oxygen into our bodies by the unconscious act of breathing. However, I really fear that is not enough, especially these days when we lead such sedentary lifestyles in front of our computers, smartphones and televisions. Our bodies are starving for oxygen. Our job is to get enough oxygen into our system so that it can function properly. The best way to get oxygen into our system is to move our bodies to the point where our heart rate is increasing. When our heart rate increases it pumps blood through our body at a faster than normal rate. The blood is carrying oxygen to the cells of our body. The more oxygen our cells get the happier they will be.

It's a sad fact but as we age the cells in our bodies start to die off. Add to that the fact that cells in our bodies are damaged by the overload of toxins found in the food we eat, the products we put on our bodies, and the air we breathe. If we sit back and do nothing, our bodies will just start to decay on us. I often see people in their 60s, 70s, or 80s who spend their days sitting in a chair. As they sit, I know that their muscles are getting weaker and weaker. It makes me sad. Old people don't get weak and fall because they are old; they get weak and fall because they don't use their muscles anymore.

Our muscles hold our bones together which in turn hold our bodies upright. Without muscles our bodies would crumble to the ground. Who wants that to happen? Not me!

So, I exercise. I want to keep the oxygen flowing through my body. I want to strengthen my heart through cardiovascular exercise and I want to strengthen my muscles through strength training. I want to support the cells of my body so they can fight against decay and disease. Our bodies are warriors for survival but we need to feed them and strengthen them so they have the energy and stamina to fight potentially harmful intruders. The process is so elementary and yet so amazingly complicated and fascinating.

More Reasons to Exercise

There are so, so many reasons to exercise, but for me, one of the major reasons I exercise is because I love the feeling I get **after** I exercise. Early in my journey I discovered how good I felt after a good workout. I loved that feeling of being alive and vibrant on the inside of my body. I kept that thought close by so that on days that I didn't want to exercise I simply asked myself if I wanted to feel great because I had exercised or did I want to feel bad because I hadn't? I simply had to remember the wonderful feeling post-workout and that was all the fuel I needed to get me out the door.

You have probably heard many fitness enthusiasts talk about the "high" or the adrenaline rush they get from working out. To be honest, I seldom get that feeling during a workout, and when I do, the feeling lasts for about two minutes if I am lucky, and then it's gone.

My favourite moments during a workout occur when I find myself accomplishing something I didn't think I could. I remember the first time I did a leg drop with a reverse crunch at Bootcamp. When the instructor demonstrated the exercise my first thought was, *"I can't do that!"* But, I did it! Then I did it again and again. I was shocked at how strong I had become without actually realizing it; I had tears in my eyes and a lump in my throat. It was a powerful moment.

I had a similar feeling one day after I had been attending yoga for close to two years. We were finishing a sequence with a seated forward fold. Basically, we were seated on our mats with our legs stretched out in front of us. The goal was to bend at the hips, folding over the legs and reaching for your toes. I have never been able to do that before. I could reach my shins but that's about as flexible as I was. On this particular day, I was seated with my eyes closed listening to the yoga teacher. As she said, *"forward fold,"* I bent forward at my hips and reached out hoping to touch my toes: no go, my toes weren't within reach. My first thought was, *"Where are my toes?"* I opened my eyes to see how far away from my toes I was, only to be shocked to see that I had actually reached past my toes! It was a crazy, exciting moment for me. Once again I had accomplished something I never thought possible.

The joy of experiencing these moments is hard to explain. It is something to be experienced through feeling not through words. These feelings, these joys, these accomplishments are there for anybody who chooses to take the path towards them. These feelings are not just for the experienced and hard-core fitness enthusiasts. These feelings are available to anybody who pushes themselves outside of their comfort zone. As a newbie to exercise, imagine climbing a set of stairs for the first time without being winded. Imagine holding plank for 30 seconds. Imagine being able to run for a whole minute. Imagine being able to swim the length of the pool without stopping. These baby steps are powerful and as important and as rewarding as reaching a *runner's high* during a 10km run. Don't underestimate the power of these first milestones. They are a strong foundation to build upon.

Many years ago when I first started to run, I literally laced up my shoes and went to the park and ran around the perimeter. Actually, I didn't run all the way, I probably ran 100 meters before I was completely exhausted and was forced to walk. However, once I caught my breath I would run again and then walk and then run. I repeated this sequence four or five times and then I went home, completely out of breath but feeling slightly triumphant because I had done it. A couple years later I signed up for a running clinic where I learned a lot about running, then I signed up for another clinic where I learned more about running, then I signed up for another clinic. I did this repeatedly until I eventually made it to the ½ marathon distance (21.1 km) and later to the marathon distance (42.2 km).

Training for my first marathon was tough. We trained through the worst winter our area had seen in about 50 years. We trained through knee-deep snow, slush, wind and rain. It was not easy but two things kept me going: 1) my dream of running a marathon and 2) the post-run feeling. Even though I am generally extremely tired and sore especially after super long runs or hill training days, I feel invigorated, alive, and strong. I wish I could bottle the feeling and sell it to people who spend their life on a couch. I wish I could give them a shot of what I feel after these long runs. But, I can't. I can only hope that my words will somehow plant a seed in their soul that will grow into a desire to move.

A while back someone asked me why I train to run such long distances if it is so exhausting. There are several reasons: 1) because it fascinates me that at my age my body can do this. 2) I love the feeling of being strong and alive and invigorated. And 3) because I will probably not leave a legacy of any great meaning, but, I can run a marathon and that is a huge accomplishment!

My hope is that you will find the motivation to lace up your shoes and get out the door and move your body. You have to start somewhere and the beginning usually starts with a first step, followed by another and then another. Each positive step forward strengthens your heart and your muscles. You will be changing old habits, forming new habits, you will see results and you will feel amazing. Treat your body as if it was your best friend and it will reward you accordingly.

One More Reason to Exercise…

If I haven't convinced you yet to start an exercise program based on the reasons that work for me: 1) your body needs as much oxygen as it can get, and 2) you will experience amazing feelings both during and after your workout, then, let me add one more reason in an attempt to convince you to start to exercise. You should exercise because of the **food**!

Yes, food and exercise are connected. My fitness journey has taught me much about food and changed my relationship with food. In my past I used to exercise so that I could eat what I wanted without guilt. I exercised because I was burning off calories that I had previously consumed. Exercise was a weight management tactic. The more I exercised the more calories I was burning which meant of course that I could eat what I wanted.

This method of weight management works great as long as you are exercising to burn the calories. However, when life gets busy, or you are tired, or you are on vacation, then the calories you are consuming are not being spent, they are being stored in your belly and on your hips.

It wasn't until 2013 when I realized that I needed to get healthy that my connection between food and exercise changed. I used to exercise so I could eat. I now eat because I exercise. There is a difference! The shift for me happened slowly and unconsciously as I plugged away learning new ways to fuel my body.

As I started to change the type of food I was eating and increased my activity level I noticed that when I ate real food with balanced nutrients that my body was able to perform better; my runs were easier, I had more energy, and I felt better. If I got lazy in the kitchen and ate whatever I could get my hands on quick and easy, I would find myself feeling sluggish during my workout with very little energy to push myself forward. This was not the feeling I was after.

My desire to feel energized during and after my workouts fuelled my desire to prepare and eat healthy meals. Because I was working out, I wanted real, tasty, energizing food. As fitness became more important in my life, I naturally changed how I looked at food. Food became fuel for my workouts instead of calories that needed to be burned. Today I rarely think about calories being burned. Of course, I know this is happening in my body, but it isn't what drives me. What drives me is a desire to feel great, to feel strong and energized, and I now know that quality food will fuel a quality workout which will make me feel great. It's a simple equation.

Exercising is now a way of life, as is eating healthy. I love to exercise and feel my body growing stronger and getting faster. I love to eat. I love food. I try new recipes all the time. I never feel deprived. I eat quality, nourishing food that satisfies my body's needs. I have never felt better. Food is a glorious thing in our lives; it is an adventure all on its own. Don't deprive yourself of all the amazing, healthy taste adventures that await you. You can bet that professional athletes don't live on grilled chicken breasts, celery sticks and cucumbers, and neither should you. Professional athletes know that they have to fuel their bodies for success.

While I am on the subject of professional athletes I want to remind you that the only thing that separates you from them is that they practice their sport over and over and over. They have chosen a life where fitness and sport is front and centre in their lives and they work diligently on developing their bodies to perform certain tasks at an elevated level. Yes, they have coaches and experts that help them reach peak performance, but at the core, their bodies are made up of the same things as yours and mine. The thing that separates them from us is their desire to be the best at what they do: that's the biggest difference.

I say this because you also have a choice when it comes to exercise and training your body to become a strong and efficient machine. The human body really is fascinating. It is capable of accomplishing amazing things. It is our brains that get in the way. Dr. Wayne Dyer says, "Change your thoughts, change your life." You may never become a professional athlete, neither will I, but our bodies deserve the same treatment and respect. Our bodies need to move and be challenged. Additionally, we deserve quality food grown and prepared in such a way that our bodies benefit physically and emotionally from it.

Ask yourself these questions:

- How do you fuel your body for success?
- Do you feed and nourish your body to the best of your ability?
- Do you exercise because you eat, or do you eat because you exercise?

- Do you love the food you eat and does your body love it too?
- Are you giving your body what it deserves and needs to be a top performer in the game of life?

Real, wholesome food can be delicious and satisfying. By nature, food is designed to fuel our bodies for success, to do all the things we need it to do. So whether you are rock-climbing, kayaking, dancing, lifting weights, pole vaulting, running, playing tennis, or jumping through the sprinkler with your toddler, give your body the best food you can. Make it a lifestyle to move your body and eat great food. Food and exercise go hand in hand. You really can have the best of both worlds.

But What Exercise Should I Do?

There is no such thing as one exercise to fit all, so to say that the best exercise is "X" would be wrong and misleading. Although I enjoy bootcamp, yoga, hiking, and biking primarily I am a runner. I am not a star runner. I will probably never make it to Boston. I did place third in my age category (50-54) one time at one of our local 10km race events. Another time I got sixth place overall in a very small 5km running event. But, that is about as accomplished as I get. Yet, I run. I have been running on and off for over 20 years. Running has been my saviour and for the most part I love it. I am someone who gets bored easily so running works for me because I can change routes, change distances, or change scenery. There is always someone new to meet and run with and of course, the weather is always different which means I need a lot of different running outfits to suit the climate. In addition, we run on all types of terrain: streets, hills, trails, and tracks.

The possibilities and variety are endless. No two runs are the same and I like that. For me, running is the best exercise.

But, running isn't for everyone. So, I am not going to answer the question I asked at the beginning of this section by saying you should run. What I will say is that I believe that the best type of exercise that you can do is one that works for you; one that you enjoy, and one that fits into your lifestyle. Exercising should be fun (as well as challenging and rewarding), and you should choose an exercise that you look forward to doing (all the time knowing that there will be days that you don't want to do it). There are many, many exercise options available to you and so a little self-analysis goes a long way. Before embarking on an exercise routine, ask yourself a few questions:

- Do you prefer to work out in the privacy of your own home? Or, do you prefer the hustle and bustle of a big, busy gym?
- Do you like to be outdoors and feel the wind and rain on your face? Or do you prefer to stay warm and dry indoors?
- Do you like to exercise alone?
- Do you prefer to exercise with a group?
- Do you enjoy team sports?
- Do you like to work out in the morning, on your lunch hour or in the evening?
- Do you like lots of variety and flexibility or do you prefer routine?
- Do you like fast-paced or slow-paced activity?

You will also want to consider your goals, or your reasons for exercising?

- Do you want to improve your cardiovascular endurance so you can walk up a flight of stairs without losing your breath? Or do you want to run a 10km race?

- Do you want to build muscle so that you look good in a bathing suit?
- Do you want to lose 5, 10, 20, 40 or 80 pounds?
- Do you want to improve your flexibility so that you can actually bend over to tie your own shoes?
- Or are you like I was and do you want to improve your overall health so that you can reduce your blood pressure, improve your quality of sleep and reduce your stress?

Whatever your goals are, some form of exercise will help you reach your goal. So ask yourself these questions and then consider a few options. Stay open and listen to what people say. Pay attention to signs that you might see. Life has an amazing way of pointing you in the right direction. But, first you must have a desire, then you must start your search, then you must pay attention to clues and finally, you must act on the clues you get.

Most importantly, don't be afraid to try new things. Step out of your comfort zone and then keep moving. There are a million different ways to move your body, so to say you can't find anything you like to do just means you haven't looked hard enough or tried enough things.

One of my beautiful sisters, Yvonne, took up aerial yoga and aerial silks at the age of 63!! She then went on to take the teacher training course!! That is amazing. She has found a new love and she is strong, fit and toned. Not only does this form of exercise develop incredible muscle strength, it also requires a lot of guts! I mean, hanging upside down from silk scarves tied to the ceiling as you twist and turn your way through a series of movements! It's amazing to me and I am so proud of my sister for all she has accomplished. Not only is she accomplished in her yoga skills, but she is also an avid golfer and a pretty darn good one at that!

If you haven't quite found a form of exercise that you love, don't worry. Just keep moving forward, keep trying new things and there will come a time where your body and your mind both click together and simultaneously say, *"Hey, I like this – this works for me!"* We are all unique individuals and our needs, wants, and desires are all different. What works for one person may not work for another, and that's okay. Actually, it's more than okay; it's how we are designed. If you join a class with a friend and it turns out that one of you loves the class and the other one doesn't, don't feel bad, don't stay stuck and don't apologize. Move on to something different. I have joined many classes by myself and ended up meeting the best people, some of whom have become really good friends. This is your journey, this is your adventure, but, you have to keep moving.

If you have looked around and tried a few things but still feel stuck or frustrated because you **just don't like to exercise**, then simply go for a walk. Walking is so simple and yet so effective. Walking will get your body moving which will get the oxygen flowing which will clear out some 'cobwebs' and allow new thoughts to enter into your mind. You can even take your walk to a new level by walking with intention. What I mean by this is: focus on your walking. Challenge yourself to hold your core tight, keep your head up and your shoulders back. Let your arms swing freely and focus on your breath. You will be amazed at how good an intentional walk feels. Your walk can be as short as two minutes to start. It doesn't matter how long you walk for. What matters is that you get out the door and do it!

As you start to feel the benefits from your short walks you will automatically want to start to take longer walks. Your body will start to look forward to the walks. Your mind will clear and amazing things may happen. You may discover that you really like walking and then decide to increase your distance which will feel so great. Maybe you'll decide to take your walk up a steep hill which will really get your heart pumping. You may even decide to incorporate a short run into your walk. Running will really get the blood and the oxygen flowing through your veins and delivered to the cells of your body – which would be a great thing!

It doesn't matter how far you go; your body will benefit from short walks as well as long walks, both physically and mentally. Why would you not want that? It's simple, it's free, it's natural, and it's oh so good for you.

The body is a fascinating thing and will take you places that you have never been before. But, you have to give it direction, you have to point the way and take a step forward. Then take another step and then another one after that. A journey is made up of thousands of steps but it starts with one.

Make It a Way of Life

No matter what you do, keep active. Incorporate fitness into your life so that it becomes as natural and necessary as eating and sleeping. Find that one thing that keeps you motivated and keeps you moving. Don't spend your life sitting in a chair. There are trails to be discovered, parks to explore, and mountains to climb. Now that I am getting older I realize more than ever the importance of exercise in my life. I now know that in order to stay active well into my 80s and hopefully 90s, I will have to continue to exercise. I will have to keep my muscles, my bones, and my heart strong. Of course I also need to keep my brain healthy as well. I know that maintaining a regular exercise routine and eating healthy food will absolutely help me on my journey.

I am grateful for the knowledge I have gained over the last several years. My wellness journey is not about looking good for an upcoming trip, or about getting in shape before a high school reunion. Fitness and well-being must be a way of life. It must be something you want to do because you know that the short-term and long-term benefits are worth it.

Many months ago I saw a picture on my cousin's Facebook page of several of my aunts and uncles. It was taken after a few of them had just finished playing a round of golf. What an inspiration! My aunts and uncles are all in their mid to late 80's and they remain active by playing golf. One of my aunts in particular has been an inspiration to me my whole life. At one point when we were very young my sister and I lived with Aunt Betty and her family. One of the things I remember most about our time together is that every morning we would turn on the TV and exercise along with Ed Allen. I remember it well, we had so much fun and most certainly a seed was planted in my soul way back then. My Aunt Betty was a huge support in my life as I grew up and continues to be an inspiration. She has remained active her whole life and is strong and vibrant well into her 80s. I have great admiration for her and I am so grateful for how she influenced my life.

Make fitness and wellness a part of your life. Make it something you want to do, not something you have to do. Enjoy yourself, have fun, and try new things. Don't be afraid of adventure and say yes as often as you can. Our world is big and beautiful. Make it a mission to get out and explore it. Make fitness and an active lifestyle a way of life. Your life will be so much more fulfilling.

Chapter 10

What We Think, Feel, Say and Do Will Come True

Over the course of my life I have read many books by some of the world's most inspirational writers on the subjects of goal-setting, visualization, positive self-talk and gratitude. Some of my favourite authors include: Norman Vincent Peale, Napolean Hill, Og Mandino, Dr. Wayne Dyer, Marianne Williamson, Rhonda Byrne, Eckhart Tolle, Louise Hay, M. Scott Peck M.D., Robin Sharma, Stephen R. Covey and Brian Tracy. These authors opened up a whole new way of thinking for me and pointed me in the direction of a happier more fulfilling life. If you have not read many inspirational books written by these or other brilliant authors, I would highly recommend that you make your way to your local book store or library and pick up a couple of motivational and inspirational books. These books will guide you through "how goal setting is so much more successful when you write your goals down", "how visualization works," "how expressing gratitude and maintaining a positive mental attitude will change your life," "how we attract what we think about" and "how we are all connected by the thread of life called Love." These subjects fascinate me and although I am far from an expert, I can share how I believe my use of these tools helped me on my wellness and weight-loss journey.

When I started, I realized I needed to tap into some of the pearls of wisdom I had learned from my readings. I knew that buried under all my stress, anxiety, self-doubt and poor decisions were tools that I could use to help dig myself out. Although I don't remember exactly what order I dug myself out of the pit I had fallen into, my journey did start by identifying my problem: I was unhealthy! I then realized what I really wanted to accomplish, so I set a goal to improve my health.

Goal Setting

The first thing you need to do is to identify what your goal is. What are you trying to accomplish? Is your goal to lose 20 pounds? Is your goal to fit into your favourite pair of jeans? Is your goal to be able to skate comfortably with your children? Is your goal to hike the Grand Canyon? What is it that you want to do? Get clear about it and write it down. The next step in Goal Setting 101 will have you then make a clear dated action plan. Think about the steps that you will need to take in order to reach your goal, and then write those steps down. The next step is to take action. The best laid plans will always fail without action. Action is the key to success.

On my journey, I kept my goal very simple: my goal was to improve my health so that I could lower my blood pressure, sleep better, have more energy and feel better. So without getting too complicated and making charts and graphs, I simply thought about what I would need to do to get healthier. Here is my action plan:

1. First and foremost, I was going to have to change what I ate and how I prepared my food so that my body received more benefits from the food I was feeding it.
2. Second, I was going to have to exercise.
3. Third, I was going to have to change my thoughts to those that matched a healthy, happy, active person.
4. The date on my goal was 'forever'. Health was something I want for the rest for my life, not just for an upcoming party or reunion.

I was reminded of the famous saying by Paul Meyer: *"If you continue to think the way you have always thought, you'll continue to get what you've always got."* I also realized that I could do all the hoping and wishing in the world, but unless I took action, nothing was going to change. Action equals results. So I began the process of improving my diet and moving my body one step at a time.

I knew that changing my thought patterns was not going to be easy because our brains just ramble on all day long about a million and ten things per minute; most of which are not even true! I likened my brain to a wild horse – continually bucking about, running away, and misbehaving. How do you control that? I imagined that slowly, slowly the wild horse would be broken, slowly it would be tamed and slowly I would take control over the wild beast; aka, my brain. But, how was I going to do that?

Affirmations

The Oxford dictionary describes *"affirmation"* as: *"Noun – 1. The action or process of affirming something. 2. Emotional support or encouragement."*
I have read about the power of using affirmations and their effect

on the subconscious mind. I have read that what you feed your mind over and over will become your reality, (if you also take some steps in the direction of you goal.) I did what the books said; I made my affirmations present, positive and to the point. When you start your affirmation with "I am" you are declaring the words that follow to be a truth about yourself. So armed with this knowledge, I made two affirmations:

1. *"I am fit, fun, and fabulous"*
2. *"I am healthy, wealthy, and wise"*

These words became my constant companions. I did not worry about how they worked, if they worked, or whether they would work for me. I just repeated these words over and over and I trusted that what I read was real: that my sub-conscious mind would start to take over and things would start to happen to lead me in the direction of my goal.

Sure enough, things started showing up to help me on my journey. I would talk to someone who told me about a book, I heard about a healthy recipe that I decided to try, I was fortunate to win the bid on a couple of silent auction items at my son's school fair that led me to yoga and bootcamp.

This stuff doesn't just happen to me. It can happen to you too. If you focus on a positive result you want to see in your life, the Universe will put events in front of you to help you. But, you have to be aware, then you have to take action, and sometimes you have to go outside of your comfort zone. You see, winning a pass to bootcamp was easy; showing up to the class was downright intimidating. After all, I was clearly the oldest person in the class, I was overweight and I was very unfit. But, I showed up anyway because my subconscious mind told me that I was *"fit, fun and fabulous!"*

Honestly, at first I did feel awkward going to those bootcamp classes. As other ladies hung around after class and laughed and talked, me, I just bolted. I was terrified to be found out. I was terrified to have to talk to anyone. What was a 50+ year old women doing coming to this class attended mostly by 20 and 30-year-olds? Oh wait! Stop the negative chatter! *"I am fit, fun and fabulous;" "I am healthy, wealthy and wise!"* I repeated this over and over and over. I was on a journey. I was literally stretching myself outside of my comfort zone. My comfort zone was boring and did nothing for my mind except let it get lazy and fall half asleep. I wanted more for myself, my mind, and my body than that. So, I practiced my affirmations until I started to believe them, even if just the smallest amount.

It's amazing to look back to my early days of bootcamp. I was so scared, but, I believe that my positive, personal, and present affirmations helped carry me through those early days. It's kind of ironic that I later became a certified fitness instructor and taught bootcamp to those same young 20 and 30-year-old ladies! I guess that's what happens when you are *"fit, fun and fabulous"* and *"healthy, wealthy and wise!"*

If you don't have an affirmation then make one; one that will carry you when you are weak, one that will pick you up when you fall, one that will put a smile on your face when all you want to do is hide and cry.

Act as If

One of the pearls of wisdom I have learned over the years is that if you want something then you need to act as if you already have it; that it already exists. Again, I don't know how it works, but, I have read enough about the concept that I believe it. On my journey I knew I wanted to be healthier, so I decided to start acting like a healthy, active person would act, and yes, it was an act sometimes! I started to really think about my choices, for instance:

- Would a healthy, active person frequently eat a hamburger, fries and a pop from a drive-thru restaurant? Or would a healthy, active person make a healthy, nutritious lunch?
  - Answer: A healthy, active person would make a healthy, nutritious lunch, so that is what I did.
- Would a healthy, active person plunk themselves on the sofa night after night and eat chips? (Okay – sometimes I still do this – work in progress!) Or would a healthy, active person get some exercise on some of those nights?
  - Answer: A healthy, active person would get some exercise, so that is what I did.
- Would a healthy, active person eat three pieces of cake?
  - Answer: No, most likely they would not, so I chose to pass on dessert many times.
- Would a healthy, active person abuse their body with too much sugar, too much junk food, too much alcohol?
  - Answer: No, a healthy, active person respects their body and wants to feed it and nurture it so that it can do all the fun activities; so I started to respect and nurture my body more.

I asked myself many, many times: *"What would a healthy person do?"* and then I made my choices accordingly. Remember, at the beginning of my journey I was not healthy, or active, therefore I had to *"act as if"* I was.

Making this change to the way I thought and subsequently acted paid off. The more that I acted as if I was already a healthy, active person; the healthier and more active I became. By choosing to focus on my goal as if I was already living my goal, I believe that I was sending a clear message to the Universe that this is who I was and the Universe replied – *"Okay!"*

I have read many spiritually based books and although I am still an infant in the scope of learning, I do believe that the Universe will give you what you focus on. I once read a story that went something like this:

> If you spend your time thinking that you "*want* to lose weight" then the Universe will give you exactly that: "a *wanting* to lose weight!" If you continually think that you "*need* to lose 30 pounds," the Universe will give you a "*need* to lose 30 pounds." In other words, you won't actually lose the weight because you are focusing and thinking about the fact that you "need" to lose the weight and the Universe says, "Okay."

Similarly, if you use language like: *"I can't run, it hurts my legs,"* then sure enough, when you try to run, your legs will hurt. Instead use language like: *"Each time I run, my legs are stronger and stronger."*

I believe very strongly that what you focus on and the language that you use will create your reality. I chose to focus on being *"fit, fun and fabulous"*, *"healthy, wealthy and wise"* and I acted like I was a fit and healthy person: I ate healthy food and I exercised. And you know what happened? I started to notice a change in my energy level. I started to feel good. My whole body started to feel energized, vibrant, and open. The cells were breathing, things were moving and shaking inside me, and I started to lose weight. For me, acting as if I was already a fit, healthy person worked.

Visualization

What part does visualization have in a weight loss or wellness program? Well, for me, it had a lot to do with it. I believe that you have to be able to see yourself as a thinner, more active, healthier person. You have to visualize yourself doing the activities that you have not been able to do as a heavier, unfit person. There are many ways of doing this. I will share a couple of techniques that worked well for me.

Many years ago I heard about vision boards or goal posters so I decided to make a vision board depicting my ideal lifestyle. I went to a thrift store and bought several old magazines. I then sat down and cut out all kinds of pictures that appealed to me in one way or another. I then glued the collage of pictures onto a 2' x 3' poster board. These pictures depict images of people doing activities that I would like to do like hiking, canoeing, and yoga. I added pictures of healthy food that looked really appealing to me: a basket of garden fresh vegetables, a little girl eating a big cob of corn, a peach tree in an orchard. I also included pictures of other things that I loved: a cottage garden, a tropical retreat, a bookcase full of books, a couple embracing, and a teddy bear hugging a teddy bear.

My goal was to create a healthy lifestyle and I wanted my collage to speak to me of exactly that, so I added words as well: *"vitality," "be bright, bold & beautiful," "loving," "world of opportunity," "food is love," "take care of your family," "this is our cottage," "kindness counts," "rediscover," "health is happiness," "fresh obsessed,"* and at the very top of my vision board is, *"Get the plan you want and take action."*

I love my vision board; for me the images speak to my heart and they make me happy. This form of visualization works for me. It's beautiful, calm and personal. When I look at my vision board I see happiness, joy and beauty: I see a healthy lifestyle! If you have never made a vision board, I would highly recommend it. It is a fun, inspirational, soul-searching exercise that will uplift you and speak to you of all the things you love and will give you a clear picture of who you are and what you desire from life. *"Ask and you shall receive."*

I believe that visualization has played a major role in my life many, many times. When my son was in elementary school I was still working full time as a sales representative. My neighbour friend and I would take turns dropping our young boys off at school and picking them up at the end of the day. We always walked our boys to the main doors in the morning and waited for them outside the doors after school. Because of my flexible work schedule, I could arrange my work appointments around pickup time, which meant that I always showed up at the school in work/business clothes. I felt awkward. I envied the other moms who wore yoga pants and running shoes and cute casual attire. Oh man! How I wished I was one of them. I often thought how lucky they were to wear such fun, active, comfortable clothes while mostly I was feeling stifled in stuffy work clothes that mostly didn't fit me well. I longed for the day when I too could dress in fun, active wear and spend my spare time exercising!

Well, you know the old saying: *"be careful what you wish for!"*

In my case, my wish came true! Not exactly how I would have chosen, but losing my job was a clear indication that I got exactly what I was thinking about and wishing for! Visualization works!

What do you think about? What do you visualize in your mind's eye? Can you see it? Can you feel it? Is it positive?

Choose your thoughts wisely and you can help create the life you dream about.

Be Good to Yourself: Show Yourself Some Love!

On my Instagram account I often use a hashtag called *#begoodtoyourself*. I can't stress how important this is. I am not talking about self-indulgent *"treats"* that we fool ourselves into believing. I am talking about genuinely taking care of yourself: nurturing yourself, making choices that support your goals, being kind in your self-talk, surrounding yourself with people and things you love. We need to take care of our bodies, our minds and our souls.

When we eat healthy, nourishing meals, we are being good to ourselves. When we choose healthy, clean, non-intoxicating drinks, we are being good to ourselves. When we exercise and spend time in nature, we are being good to ourselves. When we pursue our hobbies and our passions, we are being good to ourselves. When we spend time with people who we really love, we are being good to ourselves. When we surround ourselves with objects that express who we are, we are being good to ourselves. When we think happy, positive thoughts, we are being good to ourselves. Every time you make a choice to support your higher, healthier vision of yourself, you are being good to yourself.

Many years ago I started to write a weight loss book called *Sex Goddess or Fat Pig?* I read this over now and it makes me sad to think that I chose those words to put on paper. My message was clear: I had a choice to be either a sex goddess or a fat pig!! Wow!! That is so hurtful, so cruel and so disrespectful. My mind and my body deserve better than this ultimatum. Thankfully, that book never got past the first chapter! I now know that positive self-talk, self-love, and self-respect are important and vital components in the wellness journey.

- How do you talk to yourself?
- Are you loving, kind and respectful to yourself?
- What words do you use to lift your spirits?
- What negative, hurtful words can you start to eliminate from your self-talk?
- Are there things that you can do to be good to yourself?
- Can you surround yourself with more of the things you love?
- Can you get rid of things that you don't love?
- What one healthy habit can you implement today?
- What positive picture can you paint of your life?

We are all human beings on a journey. We all make mistakes and have setbacks. When this happens remember to be good to yourself, use kind words in your self-talk. Take care of yourself as if you were taking care of the most precious thing in the world. Self-care is not a self-indulgent act and it is not being self-centered. Self-care is vital to your well-being and the health and happiness of not only yourself, but also those around you. When you exude vitality other people will benefit: as we are all connected in this circle of life.

Gratitude

The more I read about gratitude the more grateful I become. We should teach a class in our schools about the power of gratitude. It's a magical tool that not enough people know about, or maybe they know, but they don't use it. It's easy to complain about things in our lives: we don't have enough money, our bosses are idiots, the traffic is horrible, the world is scary, and the markets are crashing....on and on and on. But, how is focusing on all the negative going to make you feel better? Answer: it's not.

But, let's face it: some days we just feel worn down and sometimes all we see and feel is pain, heartbreak, fear or sadness. When this happens to me, I dig out the magic tool called "Gratitude" and I start to write about all the things in my life that I am grateful for.

You might ask: "What does being grateful have to do with a weight loss or wellness journey?" It has a lot to do with it. In my past, as an overeater, I often turned to food to lift my spirits and make me feel better. What I learned on my journey is that there are many ways to feel better besides reaching for calorie-laden, unhealthy, fatty food: expressing gratitude is one of the ways.

Now, if I am feeling low and need something to lift my spirits I write down all the things in my life that I am grateful for and immediately I feel better. It is a magical tool that works every time. Admittedly, I did not discover this tool until after I had lost my weight and had started writing this book. Nevertheless, I believe that expressing gratitude on whatever journey you are on will help you pave a smoother path. Expressing gratitude changes bad days into good days and uplifts me in ways that no amount of chocolate, donuts, pizza, wine, or chips could ever do. It is for this reason that I believe strongly in the power of gratitude. I would like to share my first entry from my gratitude journal with you.

Gratitude Journal – Tuesday October 20, 2015

Today I start my gratitude journal because it's something I have wanted to do for a long time. I know that expressing gratitude is one of the most powerful things that anyone can do. I know from experience that being grateful for the things we have, be it people in our lives, our health, our talents, our ambitions, our mobility, our home, our jobs, our material possessions, or our goals and desires can change your day from bad to good in a few short moments. I have had bad days and I have let bad days consume me. But, I have also had bad days where a little light goes off in my head that says, "Think of things you are grateful for." Suddenly, I start to feel better. A tiny smile comes across my face and I feel uplifted. It works every time. Sometimes the uplifting feeling pulls me up high enough that I can turn my bad day right around and get busy and have a beautiful day. Other times I just feel uplifted enough to not have a bad day. But, I do know that expressing gratitude works. However, expressing gratitude when I am down is not enough. Gratitude needs to be expressed on good days and bad days. It needs to be expressed every day! Because when you express gratitude on good days, those days get elevated to great days! And who doesn't want to feel great all day long?

So today I am grateful for so many things: my home, my health, my family, my son, my husband, my dog, my friends, my fitness level, my ability and time and space to grow and learn and express myself. I am grateful to God for bringing me circumstances in my life that push me out of my comfort zone. I am grateful for everything that surrounds me. I am grateful for my book My Accidental Diet. *I am grateful for my life!!*

I share this because I think it is really important on a wellness or weight loss journey to focus on the good and the positive things in your life. It is an easy thing to do and the results are instant. The minute you think positive thoughts, you will immediately feel better.

I believe in gratitude journals and I would highly recommend that you start one. It is easy to do and costs nothing more than a couple of dollars for a notebook and a few minutes per day. Also, keep in mind that there are no hard and fast rules to keeping your gratitude journal. Sometimes I write in my journal several days in a row. Sometimes I write once a week and sometimes a few months go by without a single entry. From my experience, the more I write the better I feel. Write about anything you are grateful for: your home, your job, your health, the food in your fridge, the water from your tap, your warm bed, your new coat, your mom, your dad, your best friend, your cat, your talent, your dreams, a good book you are reading, your breakfast, your car, the flowers, the rain….just let it flow out.

Make gratitude a part of your day. It will uplift you, put a smile on your face and show you the sunny side of your life; very likely it will change your life for the better.

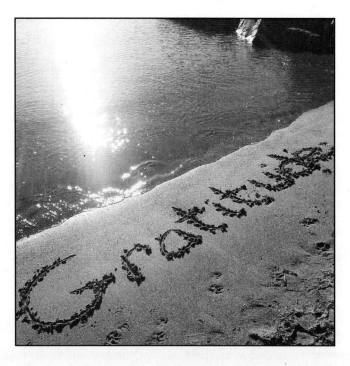

I wrote the word "Gratitude" in the sand January 1, 2016

Each person has the ability to create whatever lifestyle they want in their thoughts. The stronger your thoughts, the more believable they become. Strong beliefs lead to opportunities showing up in your life that will help you fulfill the vision in your mind. So think about your ideal life, or think about a healthy lifestyle goal that you would like to accomplish. Then spend time visualizing what that looks like.

- What are you doing?
- How do you feel?
- Where are you? Are you at home or travelling?
- Are you being physically active? Are you inside or outside?
- What are you eating? How does it taste? How does it smell?
- Are you surrounded by people and things you love?
- Or are you sitting quietly alone?
- What can you eliminate from your life that no longer serves your higher vision?
- What can you add to your life to bring more health and happiness?

Have fun thinking about your ideal, healthy life and what that looks like to you. Remember, in your mind you can have whatever you want. So go ahead, create the ideal vision and then play this vision over and over and over again. Act as if you are living that vision and the Universe will start to play along. Surround yourself with people, things, animals, plants, art, music, sights and sounds that you love. Give thanks for all the blessings in your life and watch as more blessings unfold.

Maybe your ideal, healthy vision is as simple as climbing a set of stairs without losing your breath. Focus on your vision over and over, and then climb those stairs again and again. Then one day you will realize that you have made it to the top of the staircase without losing your breath; you accomplished your goal and you will feel amazing.

Changing your thoughts, much like changing your eating and exercise habits, takes time, patience and persistence. But, if you put in the work, slowly you will start to see changes and slowly the new you will emerge from behind the blanket of doubt that shields you from the life you dream of.

My journey started by making a goal to become healthier. I created a vision of a healthy, active person. I played that vision over and over. I acted as if I was already that person by making choices that a healthy person would make. I started to treat my body with more respect and do more things that I loved to do. I gave thanks for all the blessings in my life. I created a healthier mindset and a healthier environment and I watched the pounds disappear: my vision became my reality and that was very cool!

Chapter 11

When Things Go Wrong;
Which They Will

Let's face it: on your journey you will have good days and you will have bad days, we all do! You will have days, weeks, and maybe even months where everything is falling into place and you will feel strong, motivated and invincible. It is easy to stay positive and on the right track when your stars are all lined up and everything is going your way.

But, the reality is that sometimes things go wrong. Sometimes the best laid plans fall to pieces, sometimes no matter how hard you try you can't turn things around and sometimes you feel defeated and at a loss.

Sometimes the reasons are obvious, sometimes they are not. I have had really bad days when the sun is shining and the birds are chirping and the rest of my world is happy and good, but something in me is restless, anxious, stressed, disorganized, overwhelmed, sad, lonely, frustrated, guilty, angry or hopeless. There is no particular reason for these feelings, they just creep up and show their unwelcome face and settle into my body and my mind like a virus. On these days, I want to retreat, curl up in a ball, or eat my face off. I usually do all three with great success. But, this is not a place I want to live, so I have had to learn to navigate my way through these emotions in a more positive way.

For most of my life food has been a crutch for me. When I am feeling overwhelmed, lonely, or bored, I reach for food. I want comfort and companionship and I know that the sweet and salty treats will offer me an escape from my uncomfortable emotions and so, I eat! And then I eat some more. I know that I am not the only person who does this. We all want comfort; we want to be nourished and loved. We want our stresses to leave and for a few brief moments, our feeding frenzies offer us that relief. But, the feeding frenzies provide only temporary relief, so we need to learn new ways of handling these episodes, or better yet, avoiding them all together.

In this chapter I want to share some of my stories about my feeding frenzies, partly because they are funny, but mostly because they are real life situations that many of you may relate to. Food is a glorious thing: we all love it but the reality is that we also have to limit it. In some cases you can have 'too much of a good thing.' Here are some of the food pits that I have fallen into along my journey:

Ice Cream

I eat a bowl of ice cream and the sweet, creamy deliciousness is so good; so good in fact that I have another bowl and then immediately regret it. The ice cream really isn't even that good, my stomach hurts and I don't sleep well that night.

I come across a recipe for homemade ice cream using a few simple, healthy ingredients. I make it: it's good, really good. I thoroughly enjoy it and decide that I will never have to buy ice cream again.

A few weeks pass and I am in the grocery store. My son wants ice cream. I decide to take a short-cut because what can it hurt to buy ice cream once in a while? I buy the ice cream, take it home and put it in my freezer. For the most part I stay away from the tub of ice cream, but, inevitably I start thinking about it one night and alas, I go to the freezer and scoop out a bowl full. It's good, but I need more because one bowl was not satisfying. It turns out once again that two bowls of ice cream was too much: my stomach hurts and I don't sleep well that night.

I repeat the pattern several times until one day I realize that my body is not happy when I eat two bowls of ice cream at night, so I stop doing that. My stomach doesn't hurt and I sleep better at night.

Nanaimo Bars

I enter my local grocery store. At the entrance is a large display of Nanaimo Bars. *"Those look yummy,"* I think to myself. But I am strong and healthy, so I walk right past them. A few minutes later, I find myself close to the entrance again and I walk past the display once more. This time, my mouth starts to water but, I resist the temptation and turn the other direction thinking I have won the battle against the sweet temptation.

But, alas, I have not because a few minutes later I am drawn towards the Nanaimo Bars again. But, this time my hand reaches towards the pile and a tray of those delicious little treats ends up in my grocery cart. I tell myself that I am buying them for my husband. I smile because I have just justified this heavenly purchase.

Later, as I unpack my groceries the Nanaimo Bars start calling my name, I ignore them. Then they start singing to me! How can I resist that? I decide that it would be okay to have just one. *"Oh my, that was so sweet and delicious!"* I immediately reach for another – what could it hurt? *"Oh boy – what have I done? I am so stupid!"* I suddenly realize that I will now have to suffer the consequences of these two Nanaimo Bars for hours! My stomach hurts! I feel gross! What was I thinking?

The next day the chocolate goodness starts calling my name again. But, this time, I decide to outsmart the deliciously deceptive bars. I know from experience that two pieces would make me feel ill, so I control myself and eat only one and a half pieces! How smart was that? Nope!! Big mistake, I feel like crap again.

By day three and four I have it figured out; if I only eat one piece of Nanaimo Bar, I won't feel like crap and so that is what I do. By day five it hits me: what the heck am I doing? Why am I eating these bars? I had probably consumed thousands of calories, hundreds of grams of fat and sugar and countless toxins! All for a few brief moments of creamy, chocolaty deliciousness in my mouth. It's not worth it! I quit! I cut up the Nanaimo Bar and put it in the freezer. I should have put it in the garbage, but, I am not there yet.

I know from repeated experience that what my body wants is real food. I finally listen. I know that sweet treats are a simple pleasure in our lives but there has to be a better way. There has to be a healthy, natural, sweet-treat option that I can make and enjoy even more than those store-bought Nanaimo Bars. Yes, indeed there is. The next day, I make some healthy energy balls that are rich, delicious, fulfilling and made with ingredients that my body will benefit from. I got the recipe from a friend of mine Patti Fleury, who is a holistic nutritionist in Calgary and author of *Life After Crohn's*. With Patti's permission I share her recipe on page 221.

These energy balls are delicious and will rival any store-bought Nanaimo Bar, any time, any day. It is a good idea to make these and freeze them so that when your sweet tooth lights up, you will have a healthy, sweet treat to satisfy it....guilt and gut-ache free. The lessons and the learning continue.

Butter Tarts

I am tired, I have too much going on, and I haven't been sleeping well. Suddenly, my brain makes a suggestion to me: *"How about some butter tarts?"* My body perks up: *"Butter tarts?! – oh my – now that sounds good!!"* The other side of my brain says: *"No Rhonda, don't do it."* Butter-tart brain yells back: *"YES Rhonda, do it!! You will be so happy; they will make you feel better! They will pick you up and man oh man, do they taste good!"* My mouth starts to salivate. I hear my fit brain quietly whisper: *"But, Rhonda, you will feel awful."* But, the voice is so quiet because butter-tart brain is bouncing around with happiness and joy and the rest of my body joins in the party.

I get in my vehicle and drive to the store. I check my mouth to make sure the saliva isn't dripping out of the corner of my mouth. I get to the butter tarts and they are smiling at me. I grab a six-pack and put it in my cart. I buy a few other things that I may or may not need to make it look like I didn't just come to the store for butter tarts – because that would look bad.

I get through the till and then start walking towards my vehicle at a slightly faster than normal pace. I can barely contain myself as I place the bag of goodies on the passenger seat beside me. Before I am even out of the parking lot I have single-handedly opened the package of butter tarts and sank my teeth into the sweetness: my mouth is dancing and fireworks are going off in my brain. The goodness explodes and sends happy vibrations throughout my body and then yells for more.

So, I reach for another morsel of divine pleasure and pop it in my mouth. The pleasure lasts for about 30 seconds as the sweetness swirls around my mouth, but then I swallow and immediately my brain wakes up as I realize what I have just done. I feel sick to my stomach: *"Oh how stupid of me! What have I done?"* Now I will have to suffer the consequences for hours as my body deals with the overload of sugar, fat and toxins that I have just mindlessly devoured. I feel remorse and sadness that I have disrespected my body so badly. I think: *"What is wrong with me? When will I learn?"* My body deserves better than this.

I spend the next few hours sad and confused as to why I let this happen over and over again. My body is my vehicle. I need to take care of it. I need to treat it with the utmost respect. I need to fuel it and love it and in return it will reward me with health and vitality. I messed up, but, I will not dwell in the negative patterns. Instead, I will make positive choices going forward....or at least I will do my best.

Wheat

The last couple of weeks have been crazy. I have been eating very poorly, but, sometimes life gets too busy and too crazy and I end up eating whatever I can put my hands on. For me this meant pizza, ready-made sandwiches, pasta, and take-out Chinese food! You get the picture. My belly is not happy and I haven't been sleeping well. I know from my past three years of healthy eating that wheat is not my friend. When I eat wheat repeatedly I end up looking like I am five months pregnant. I woke up this morning craving poached eggs on toast (there is the wheat craving again!). But, I know I have to break the wheat cycle because it will take me nowhere very quickly; I need to kick wheat in the butt and regroup.

So, instead of toast, I opt for a cauliflower/quinoa crust that I have in the freezer. I pop it in the toaster, and then proceed to make some poached eggs. I layer the crust with pesto, spinach and top with the eggs. I serve this with a side of salsa and avocado slices. This tastes so good and I know my body will be much happier with all the nutrients and goodness that this breakfast will offer me. I also know that my body will reward me with lots of energy and a much flatter belly. Finally, I know that my body won't keep my up at night as it tries to deal with an onset of food that doesn't serve me well. Still learning!

Post-Marathon Binge

On May 9 2017, I completed my first marathon (42.2 km). It was hard work and took months of training and preparation. On the day of the race I felt ready; I knew I had done everything that I could to prepare. We had trained through snow, wind, rain and sleet. We did hill training, speed training and long, slow distance training. I had been eating good, healthy meals. I was hydrated and I was rested. I anticipated that the run would take me about five hours but, I wasn't as concerned about my finish time as I was about just finishing the race upright and with a smile on my face.

It was a beautiful day in Vancouver the day of the race and we started out slow and steady. I made several stops along the way; I had family members to hug, I had to take pictures, I had to stop for a snack half way through the race, and I had to go to the bathroom a few times. In the end, the race took me five hours and 31 minutes. I tried not to be bothered by the time knowing all along that I was not racing against the clock and that I really had enjoyed some very special moments in the race like seeing my brother not once, not twice, but three times along the route – this was a miracle and I loved every second of our time together. My brother had been dealing with the after effects of a bone marrow transplant due to a leukemia diagnoses two and a half years prior. So seeing him out and about on race days was a gift. He even ran with me for a couple hundred feet; this was special indeed.

But, truthfully, the runner in me was very disappointed with my time: I thought I had trained harder, I thought I was prepared, I thought I was fit and strong. So, when I finished so far at the back of the pack I was really disappointed and I started to over indulge.

At first it was the celebratory dinner and wine followed by movie nights with chips and chocolate.

Another night shortly after the race we ordered pizza and had more wine.

Then more chips and I actually ate a couple of sandwiches (which I rarely eat) because I didn't care.

I went through the drive-thru and ordered a donut and stuffed it in my face.

I started to crave chocolate so when I got a huge chocolate bar on Mother's Day, I promptly stuffed that in my face too.

I went to Costco and was tempted to sample a delicious looking lemon cake, it was amazing and I bought one. Within three days the cake was gone.

I ate like this for several days, each day feeling worse and worse. My stomach was bloated, I had stomach cramps, my body felt shaky and I had constant cravings. I knew exactly what was wrong and yet I wasn't prepared to do anything about it until lunch on the ninth day of my out-of-control feasting.

By some grace, when I went to my fridge that day looking for something delicious to eat, a little voice inside my head said, "Eat a salad!" PHEW! I knew I was going to be okay: my body had had enough and my brain started to call the menu. I made a salad and enjoyed it thoroughly.

Over the next couple of days, I made a point to take back the control and before long I was once again eating like a healthy, sane person and fuelling my body with foods fitting a marathon runner.

I share these stories to illustrate that my eating habits are far from perfect and that my journey has not been along a straight paved highway. I have been through many valleys, hit many speed bumps and potholes, and had to navigate my way around my emotions that send me to the fridge looking for comfort and companionship. I also share these stories with the hope that you recognize yourself or that you can possibly relate to my stories. I know that I am not alone on my journey and neither are you. I have recognized that filling my body with excessive food or food full of false promises will not make me feel better, and it won't make you feel better either.

So what can we do to make ourselves feel better when we are feeling vulnerable and weak, besides jumping into a feeding frenzy?

Without laying out a 12-step plan to controlling unhealthy eating binges; I would like to share three simple ideas that worked for me on my journey. .

1. I started to really pay attention to how I felt after eating food that was either too much or unhealthy. What I found was that although I loved the 30 seconds of deliciousness of chocolaty creamy Nanaimo Bars on my tongue, the fallout from the indulgence most often led to regret, disappointment, ill-feelings, sleeplessness, suffering, cramps, remorse and sadness, none of which are feelings that I was hoping for. I started to focus on

how I wanted to **feel**, and then made my decisions accordingly. I noticed that the more I said *"no"* to unhealthy dessert bars, cookies, donuts, tarts, chips, cake, pizza, and wheat, the better I felt. Not only did my belly not hurt, but, I felt empowered. In short, saying *"no"* made me feel great! And feeling great is my goal.

2. I had to identify the emotions or trigger points that sent me over the edge or made me make choices that I later regretted. For me, my biggest trigger points are boredom, frustration, being tired and feeling overwhelmed. I realized that food was not going to take away the boredom – doing something takes away boredom. Food does not take away frustration – but communication and organization usually do. Food does not make me feel rested – but getting enough sleep certainly helps me feel better. Food does not make me feel less overwhelmed – but taking steps to complete projects always takes the pressure off. You will have different trigger points than I do. So, go ahead and ask yourself: *"What pushes you to the fridge?"* Then ask yourself: *"Will food help solve this problem?"* Hopefully you will see that it won't, and then you can ask yourself: *"What can I do to take away or solve this stress that is pushing me towards food?"* Then make a positive, healthy choice that will help solve the problem. Oh, and please, please don't blame other people. How many of us have had a disagreement with a co-worker, parent, friend or spouse and headed to the fridge to *'show them!'* The only person you are hurting is yourself, so please, don't sabotage yourself because someone else has been a jerk towards you. Love yourself, hold your head high and do what is BEST for your body. You deserve better – just keep telling yourself that. The only trigger

point that should push you to the fridge is a genuine feeling of hunger because your body needs nutrition to keep going. Real nutrition: protein, healthy carbohydrates and healthy fats. The other trigger points that send you searching for food will not be solved by food and if it tries to tell you otherwise, it is lying!

3. I recognized that there were times where my cravings would kick in and I couldn't focus on how I would feel if I succumbed to the tasty temptation and I didn't have the patience or fortitude to work through my emotions. After falling face first into the fridge several times, I realized that I needed a plan to help me out of those nasty downward spirals that I found myself in from time to time. So, when I was feeling calm, happy and healthy, I made a list of several things I could do to distract me and steer me away from the pending disaster. Here is my list:

   a. Make a cup of herbal tea and serve it in a fancy tea cup. (This is a special treat and your taste buds will be stimulated.)

   b. Sew or do some other hobby. (Sewing is therapeutic for me, I find it calming and creative and it keeps my mind focused on a special project, it keeps my fingers busy, and it keeps my body out of the kitchen.)

   c. Take a bath. (I like to use Epsom salt, essential oils, and bubbles. Your body will love the pampering.)

   d. Go for a walk. (Just getting out of the house does wonders at getting my mind off food.)

   e. Clean a closet or drawer or just go try on clothes in your closet as if you are shopping. (I like to try on new combinations of clothes that I haven't thought about before. I then take pictures of the combinations. This comes in handy on days when I can't figure out what to wear. I can then look back at the pictures and come up with a great new look.)

f. Make some healthy muffins or cookies. (Sometimes the action of working with the food and smelling the fresh baked goodies is enough to satisfy me and keeps my hands and my mind busy.)

These are some of the activities that work for me – most of the time! And when they do work, I *feel* great (there is that *"feeling"* again!), and I *feel* proud and strong. Admittedly, sometimes I don't make it to my list and I eat two pieces of pie and then grab a bag of chips! I usually end up with a stomach ache and I usually don't sleep so well on those nights. But, hey, I do the best I can. Life is life, it's not perfect and neither am I. I wake up the next morning and move forward.

I am not 100% there; I don't think I ever will be. From what I have learned about the brain is that there are pathways of behaviour and beliefs that get etched in our brains that will most likely always exist. But, what I have also learned is that we can mend those pathways and create new ones. So, I eat healthy food and I exercise and I do this over and over again. I do this to create new healthy-habit pathways in my brain. But, I also do it because I want to feel good. Most of the time I know that no amount of ice cream, butter tarts, chips, wine, chocolate, pizza or lemon cake is going to make me feel better. What is going to make me feel better is a salad and a run.

So, I make my choices accordingly, I choose to exercise, I choose healthy food and as a result I mostly feel great. But, when I fall (which I do), I get back up, I forgive myself for my weaknesses, I give thanks for the progress I have made, and I slowly get back on the healthy highway. Living in regret and remorse is not a healthy choice and does not support my mission, so I am not going to stay in that place.

I know how to make positive healthy choices and so that is what I do; one decision at a time.

When Exercise is challenging

So far in this chapter I have shared stories with you about my misadventures with food and learning to pick myself up after I had fell face first into the proverbial box of donuts. But, I can't complete this chapter without sharing a few stories about the challenges I have faced along my road to fitness. Just like my eating habits, my fitness habits and routines have been anything but smooth sailing. I have had to start over many times. I have had many struggles along the way, I have had setbacks, obstacles to overcome, injury to recover from, and pure laziness to battle. But, somehow I always find my way back to fitness because I know deep down that I am a much happier person when I am fit.

Chances are at some point you will have your own fitness struggles to overcome or you may have to totally start over because life has thrown you completely off course. When this happens, know that you are not alone. I share the following stories with you in the hopes that they will provide inspiration and reassurance that setbacks, obstacles, and starting over are all part of the fitness journey. Additionally, I hope that you see that these setbacks are also the building blocks of a strong physical foundation. I am reminded of the saying, *"When the going gets tough, the tough get going."* Obstacles will make you stronger and discovering your true strength to overcome these obstacles is a gift. Learning to pick up the pieces after things go wrong will become part of your journey, just as they were part of my journey.

September 2009 – "The Fender Bender"

I had been running on and off for about 10 years by now. I had finally worked my way up to the half marathon distance which is 21.1 kilometers. We were just a couple weeks away from our goal race which was the Victoria half marathon. We had put in 95% of the work, now all we had to do was rest, hydrate, eat healthy, and get in a few shorter runs. I felt ready and my goal was to run the 21.1kms in two hours and 15 minutes.

Then, in a split second, my plan was thrown out the window: I was rear-ended while sitting in my van at a stop light. *BANG*, my head snapped forward as I realized I had been hit from behind. It turned out that the damage to my vehicle was minimal, but, my neck and shoulders did not fare so well.

Initially I did not realize the damage that had been done so I made the decision to continue on with my plans to run the race, at the same time making a deal with myself that I would take the race slow and easy. I walked a lot and in the end it took me two hours and 42 minutes to finish the race. I was very disappointed but I knew I had done the best I could in spite of my injury.

The injury to my neck and shoulders took many months of chiropractor treatments, physiotherapy and acupuncture treatments. During this time, my chiropractor referred me to a personal fitness trainer who specialized in rehabilitation. He also advised me to quit running until the damage done to my neck and shoulders was repaired. This was not good news for someone whose only form of exercise was running! But, I was desperate to heal my injury so I listened to his advice and I quit running and I started to see the personal trainer who worked with me twice a week for about a month. The results were awesome. He focused on helping me build the smaller muscles that support my major running muscles; he helped strengthen my neck and shoulder muscles. We worked on my core strength and in the end the therapy worked great. Slowly, I started running again, one block at a time.

By May 2010 I was ready to run my first 5km event.

Then my sister convinced me to run with her in the 14km *Coho Run* in Vancouver in September 2010. Because of my injury and lack of running, I doubted my ability to run that distance, but because my sister was coming from out of province with her family, I signed up. I also made the decision not to push myself too hard and that I would walk when needed and that I would definitely walk up any hills. Besides, the *Coho Run* is a beautiful run that starts at Kitsilano Beach, winds along English Bay Beach, through Stanley Park, over the Lions Gate Bridge, and ends at Ambleside Park in West Vancouver. This run seemed fun and doable, I was apprehensive but excited.

As we started the drive into Vancouver on race day a light rain was falling. By the time we got to Vancouver, it was pouring. My sister did not have a rain jacket, so I gave her mine: my husband gave me his rain jacket and off we went in the pouring rain. I started off slow and steady as planned. My sister was joined by a friend of hers and they were faster than I was, so before too long, I was running on my own. The run was fairly easy along the flat waterfront route. I took it easy and walked several times. However, as we entered Stanley Park we had some pretty decent elevation to climb. It was tough, but I took my time and walked up the hills as planned.

The next part of the run was crossing the Lions Gate Bridge. By this stage, we were at least 10km into the run and I was tired and soaked to the bone. Water was running down my back, down my front, up my sleeves and squishing between my toes. I should have just gone without the rain jacket for all the good it did me. As I approached the bridge deck I could see the gradual climb to the crest. I started to walk as planned, but something happened: suddenly a determination, a hidden strength, an *"I can do this"* spirit took over my body and I started to run: there was no way I was walking across that bridge!

I ran the entire length of the bridge; up to the crest and down to the base on the other side. It was magical. I felt like a woman on fire: unstoppable, strong and powerful. I felt like singing from the depths of my soul, *"I am woman, hear me roar!"* I was full of emotion and joy as I ran across that world famous bridge. The elevation didn't stop me, the rain didn't stop me, my lack of running didn't stop me; in fact, they fuelled me. To this day that run is one of my absolute favourite memories. I was not prepared for the distance, I was not prepared for the weather, and I was not prepared for the elevation. But, mostly, I was not prepared for how powerful and magical a running experience could be. I never knew how strong I was, and so I say to you as well:

"You will never know how strong you are until you try."

Don't let the weather stop you from reaching your goals and don't let an injury stop you from picking up the pieces and carrying on. In the end, I believe that my injury was a gift. Had I not gone to the personal trainer who worked to heal my neck, strengthen my supporting muscles and develop my core strength, I would have never been able to finish the race as strong as I had. Of course, I didn't realize the gift I was given until several injuries and several years later. Again, each obstacle is a building block in the foundation of your health and wellness.

Chapter 11

January 2011 – "Back on the Road – or so I Thought"

After the **Coho Run** in September of 2010, I felt refuelled and excited
to be back on the road again. In January of 2011 I sat down and made
my list of running goals:

Apr 17	Sun Run	Vancouver	10km
May 29	Run For Water	Abbotsford	10km
June 26	Scotia Bank Half	Vancouver	21.1km
Sept 11	Coho Run	Vancouver	14km
Oct 9	Marathon	Van/Vic/Kelowna	42.2km
Nov 6	Marathon	New York City	42.2km

My biggest goal was to run a marathon. I knew I needed to make my
goal race a big deal so that I could keep myself motivated and on track.
I laid out my whole year including training clinics and goal races. I
managed to find a group from North Vancouver who were training for
the **New York City Marathon**. I paid to join the group, I paid for my
entry into the race, I paid a deposit on the flight and accommodation
and then I started my marathon training. Running in New York City
was an epic goal and I was pumped.

My year started out pretty much as planned. I ran in the **Vancouver
Sun Run** as planned. I ran the **Run For Water** in Abbotsford as
planned. I skip the **Scotia Bank Half** because 1) I wasn't quite ready to
run the distance and 2) I was saving my money for the marathon trip.

In July of 2011 I had started my marathon training clinic. I was just
over three months away from my goal race when one Sunday we were
out for about a 16km run when suddenly my knee started experiencing
a lot of pain. It got so bad that I was forced to stop. We were out in the

country so the run leader called her husband to pick me up. (I am not sure where my husband was!) I ended up taking a week off running to rest my knee and by the following Sunday I was rested and ready to run again. Things were going quite good. We were about 16km into our 18km run when once again my knee gave out. This time I was determined to finish the distance so I ended up limping my way back to my vehicle. I realized that I was going to have to get my knee looked at because obviously rest was not the only thing it needed.

The problem was diagnosed as "Patella Femoral Pain Syndrome." Basically, my knee cap had been pulled out of alignment due to muscle imbalance in my leg. So, back to physiotherapy and chiropractor I went. I was advised to take three weeks off running!! *"NO! I can't do that; I am training for a marathon!"* I was at the point in the program where if I took three weeks off, I would never catch up. I was once again faced with the decision to run, or not run. I chose to cancel my trip to New York City and along with it went my dream of running a marathon (or so I thought). It was devastating to me and for a while I stopped running.

2012 – 2013 – More Injuries, Less Running

At the time of my marathon training, I was convinced by a lady I was running with that the reason for my knee pain was because I was running in the wrong shoes. She convinced me to buy into the idea that minimalist shoes were better for people's feet because they forced the foot muscles to develop better than if my feet were cushioned in a traditional running shoe. What she said made sense to me so I decided to give them a try; I bought a pair of minimalist shoes and started running again.

This experiment turned out to be a disaster. I ended up with "Plantar Fasciitis." This is a condition where the muscles in the bottom of your feet get stressed and cause pain in your arch and heels. Any runner knows that this condition is painful, running is very difficult (if at all), and the only thing you can do is roll it out on a massage ball or frozen water bottle and let it rest, which of course is easier said than done because we use our feet everyday just to walk, meaning that the muscles never really get the rest they need and the injury takes a long time to heal.

Because of my newest injury I only ran one 5km race in 2012: I did the 5km **Run For Water** with my nine-year-old son. My time was 38 minutes and 40 seconds (not very fast), his time was 32 minutes and 29 seconds. I insisted he stay close to me for the duration of the race but, he wouldn't have any part of it! My son had discovered running and he liked to challenge me.

One evening in January 2013, my family and I were out for a walk. We came to a hill and my son challenged me to race him up the hill. Of course I can do that! As I said, *"On your mark, get set...."* I took off up the hill. He quickly passed me – I was laughing too hard, at least that's my excuse for letting a nine-year-old beat me! Then suddenly something hit my leg from behind. It felt like a speeding rock had hit my calf; the pain was instant and really sharp. My first reaction was to blame my husband and son for throwing a rock at me which was ridiculous because they were ahead of me. (We laughed about that one for years – yes they were so talented that they could throw a rock and have it boomerang back the other way!) Anyway, I managed to make my way up the rest of the hill and I limped home one more time.

By the next day my foot and calf were black and blue and very swollen. I was having a hard time walking. I made my way to a walk-in medical clinic. The doctor suspected I had torn my calf muscle and sent me for an ultrasound. Sure enough, that is exactly what happened. This injury couldn't have come at a worse time as we were leaving the following week for a trip to Disney World and a four-day cruise to the Bahamas. Since I could barely walk on my leg, the only way I was able to navigate my way through airports, Disney World and a cruise ship was with the use of a wheelchair. This turned out to be a bit of a silver lining because, being in a wheelchair meant priority boarding and skipping all the long line-ups at Disney World and on the cruise ship!

After this recent injury, I was left shaking my head, trying to figure out what was wrong and why I was continually getting injured: first the fender bender, then my knee blowout, then plantar fasciitis, and now a torn calf muscle. I decided that my body was trying to tell me something: *"running was too hard on me and I shouldn't do it."* The only running I did in 2013 was the **Run For Water** 5km race with my son, mostly because I wasn't comfortable letting him run by himself. Of course, he didn't stick by my side and he beat me again. After this race, I didn't run for two years, not because my son beat me again, but because I felt like I was beat by running; I felt defeated.

March 2013 – New Challenges, New Directions

At the beginning of my book, I spoke about losing my job in March of 2013. I was not healthy and knew I had to change many things. I had hung up my running shoes but knew I wanted and needed some form of exercise. Through a series of events, I found my way to bootcamp class. This was a new, fun, and excellent workout. I felt rejuvenated and I started to see some results from all the hard work. Within a few months I was inspired by one of my sisters to take some fitness education classes. I took a series of courses which lead me to my group fitness and personal trainer certification in May 2014. For about a year or so after that I taught bootcamp classes and did one-on-one personal training with a couple of friends. I enjoyed teaching fitness and at the time it seemed to fit well into my life.

However, as life changes, I found myself once again struggling to balance several things in my life. For a number of reasons I had to make the decision to give up my certification which meant that my career as a fitness instructor was short lived, but the experience was invaluable to my fitness journey.

Although I did not teach for too long, I did continue to attend bootcamp classes as a participant. I learned a lot from the process. Mostly I learned to listen to my body. I had to face the fact that I wasn't 20 years old, (or 30 or 40....) and that I had very sensitive shoulders and neck. I had to learn to modify many of the exercises and rest when necessary. I had no choice but to accept my body's limitations and workout within them.

When we learn to listen, our bodies will tell us what works and what doesn't. Sometimes we have to stop doing a certain exercise, sometimes we have to modify or adjust. Sometimes we have to just do something different all together. I believe these challenges are all part of the process for us wanna-be amateur athletes. Who knows, someday in the distant future I may have to stop running. When and/or if that that time comes, I will certainly mourn the loss of my beloved friend "running", but I won't sit and cry too much. I will find something new to do: some new way to exercise my body. I will never stop exercising, it just feels too good! Change is inevitable, so we might as well accept the changing tides and make the most of it.

A while back I was speaking with another one of my beautiful sisters.

At the time, she was in an exercise slump. She had been going regularly to Bickram Yoga and she had loved it. But, most recently she had lost her motivation and desire to go. She expressed her concerns that she didn't know what to do because she didn't want to give up on yoga the way she had given up on other diet and exercise programs! I could tell from her tone and her words that she was sad, disappointed and frustrated with her changing relationship with yoga. This made me sad too because she didn't see that it's okay to change things up. It's not about giving up; it's about giving way to something new in her life. She didn't see the potential in the new and undiscovered. She only saw the loss of the yoga. Life evolves and grows; we are supposed to move forward, not stay in one place.

If you find yourself tired of yoga, or any other activity, for Heaven's sake – do something different! Don't feel bad, don't feel like a failure. Be kind to yourself, give yourself permission to grow and experiment and experience as many things as possible until you find out what works for you. Don't apologize for trying a bunch of new exercise options; our bodies and our minds love being challenged and stretched. You are doing yourself a huge favour by trying new things. I have done this over and over again. True, I will never become an expert at any one thing, and I am perfectly okay with that!

Fall 2015 – Picking up the Pieces

Sometimes we have to pick ourselves up after a slump or an injury or an illness. I share the following story with you about picking myself up after the summer of 2015.

Chapter 11

September 15, 2015

Dear Diary

I can't believe how awful I feel. I know that I have let my fitness level slide over the summer. But, I thought that the hikes I was doing and the walks were keeping me fit enough. It's true that those things were good for me. But, I see clearly now that my fitness level slipped further than I had realized. Last Wednesday I went back to bootcamp for the first time since early July. I knew that I would hurt, but I decided that the circuit class was a great reintroduction for my body. I made it through the class okay, not great, but okay. Two days later I was so sore I could hardly walk! I limped and whined my way through the rest of the week!

But, besides the sore muscles I have seen clearly that the lack of exercise has also affected my mood, my drive, my sleep, my metabolism, my patience, my joy and my happiness. I blew up at Conner two nights ago. I blew up at Lyndon last night. That is not who I want to be or how I want to behave. I am so sad and disgusted with myself. Why did I not handle the situations differently? Why did I lack compassion, patience, and understanding? Why was my fuse so short? As I lay awake in bed last night it came to me that my lack of exercise has affected me in more ways than one. I know that when I initially got fit that I slept better, I was happier, more loving, more understanding, not as sad and depressed. It came to me that the thing I need to do to get back to a happier place is to get back to the level of fitness I had prior to summer. Those happy hormones need to run through my veins again. I need oxygen and life and energy to flow through every cell of my body again. I knew that exercise made me feel better and now I have just had a summer of relaxation and fun to remind me. I guess my body is screaming at me as much as I was screaming at Lyndon last night. I am sorry! I am sorry to my husband. I am sorry to my son. Heck, I am even sorry to the neighbours who probably heard me yelling and crying like a woman gone mad. But, mostly I am sorry to my body for ignoring you over the summer and for taking you for granted. You do so much for me. The least I could do is give you the time and energy that you need to stay happy, balanced, energetic and loving. Please forgive me!! I will ease you back into fitness. Today's walk and 15-minute workout felt great. Tomorrow we will go to bootcamp again. You deserve it! I love you my beautiful body! Be patient with me, sometimes I forget!

Two days after this entry in my journal I made my way back to running. On September 17, 2015 I walked into my local running store and signed up for the "Learn to run 5km" clinic. Although I had done next to no running in the previous three years, there was something in my soul that called me to try again, and so I did.

Starting over at the 5 km distance was a humbling experience. My ego wanted to jump in and proclaim that "I am a half marathon runner and I was training for the **New York City Marathon.**" Instead, I joined the beginner runners and ran for one minute, then walked for two minutes, and then we repeated this six times. I was keeping my promise to myself and my body.

Starting over that day reminded me of a conversation I had had some time prior with a friend. I was trying to convince her not to look at "starting over" as a bad thing, but more as a continuation of something you have done in the past. I was really contemplating the idea of "starting over" and on September 18 I wrote this in my journal:

You will never lose what you did. You will never lose the fact that you ran 10 km five years ago. You will never lose the fact that you went to kickboxing class three times. You will never lose the games of baseball you played or the miles that you walked your dog. You can't lose that stuff so why do people insist on continuing to negate all of the positive that they have done in the past by saying that they have to start over. It's not starting over. You are simply picking up where you left off. Your memory won't forget what you did, and neither will your body. Oh sure – your muscles will be sore but before you know it you will be feeling stronger, more alive and energetic, and then you will remember, really remember, and it will be like you never quit: you just keep going!

We pick up where we left off and we carry on in one direction or the other. Life is a beautiful maze. We can stand in fear not knowing where to turn next or we can wander freely, sometimes going around in circles, sometimes wandering the same path, sometimes discovering a whole new path to wander, but each time can be a different experience if we let it be. There is a beautiful musical line in the Mary Poppins story: *"Anything can happen if you let it."*

2016-2017 – My Fitness Journey Continues

Upon completing my 5km running clinic, I joined the 10km clinic. During this clinic I met Shelley; she would become not only a dear friend, but a big supporter of me as I was writing this book. Most runners know that our love of running is not just about the physical exercise of running. It becomes about the people, the sense of community and the joy of sharing endless miles of great conversation. We pick each other up, laugh, share stories and feed off each other's energy. Shelley came as a gift to me and I am so grateful.

We ran in the 2016 10km *Vancouver Sun Run* together. We joined the half marathon clinic together. We ran the *Hypothermic Half*

Marathon together in January 2017. We then immediately joined the marathon clinic which was led by her very enthusiastic and passionate triathlete son. Without Shelley, her son and the rest of the clinic members, I don't know if I would have been able to complete the training. The support and togetherness was what made the difference between make or break! I share the following story with you:

Training Through the Worst Winter Ever

I am training for a marathon through the winter. It's the worst winter we have had in 50 some years – just my luck! But, we have a large group of like-minded souls who all have a goal to run a marathon in the spring, so we have no choice but to train in the winter through the snow, the sleet, the rain, and the wind. We train Sunday mornings, as well as Wednesday and Thursday nights. Sunday morning runs are tolerable. We run through lots of snow and some slushy sections; our feet get soaking wet, but, the scenery is beautiful. There are snow-covered trees, fields, and mountains in the distance. Sunday mornings are good. But, Wednesday and Thursday nights are usually a different story; they are tough, really tough! I start most of them in a really bad mood. I am even a little angry: "Why does the weather have to be so awful?" It's cold, it's slushy or icy on the roads, and the wind and snow are blowing in our faces. It is downright miserable outside and I am miserable inside. All I want to do is stay home where it is warm and dry, curled up in a blanket to watch a movie with my family. But, that is not going to get me across the finish line at the marathon. The only thing that will get me across the finish line is if I practice and persevere, so I reluctantly get dressed in layers of clothes and I show up to run club. To my amazement, most everyone else shows up too. We show up because our goals and our dreams are bigger than the obstacles the weather throws in our face.

It's not easy getting started, we are cold and initially our muscles are not very happy with us, but we continue to put one foot in front of the other. Gradually, we start to warm up and our bodies start to recognize what we are doing. Before long we have covered a kilometer, then another and then another. By about kilometer three my mood is starting to improve and I am warm. We run on. We even laugh a bit because it's actually kind of fun running in such ridiculous conditions! Who does that? WE DO! – as we high-five each other at the completion of our run. What a great run! We did it! Woohoo! We stretch and then head home. The hot shower feels amazing. I am so happy that I went for a run. I feel great! It wasn't even that cold – actually I was warm for most of the run! All is good and my body and my mind are very happy. I am so grateful that I chose to run. I am grateful for my running buddies who put up with my grumpiness. I am grateful for the shared laughter and joy at completing each run. They are the reason I show up even when I don't want to. We fuel each other, we care, and we support each other's goals. I feel so blessed and I always feel better after a run – always! My runs are a gift to me and in the end, I am grateful for every one of them.

I hold on tight to the post-run thoughts and feelings because I know I will need the memory of those wonderful feelings to get me out the door on the next cold and miserable evening run.

During our training there were many days and nights that we struggled to complete our training, but, we stuck together. The weather even forced us indoors onto treadmills a couple of nights. If you have ever run 16kms on a treadmill you will know how brutally boring it is. Thank God for friends to share these experiences with. Those runs built our strength, our endurance and our determination.

Eventually the weather started to improve just in time for our extra-long training runs. But, as our runs grew longer, my doubt started setting in. Then one night I had a dream: my friend Shelley and I crossed the finish line at the marathon holding hands with our arms raised in the air. I shared this dream with Shelley and you know what happened? In spite of all the obstacles we had to overcome during our training, the pain that Shelley experienced in her knee for at least half the run and the incredible fatigue we endured, we did it; we crossed the finish line at the *Vancouver BMO Marathon* in five hours, 31 minutes and 32 seconds. We were holding hands and our arms were raised in the air.

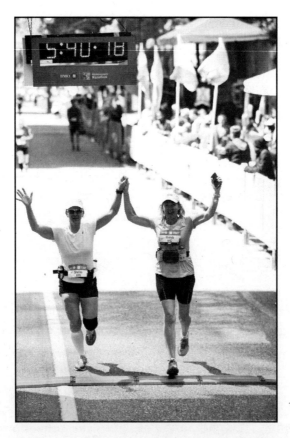

Finishing the marathon was a dream come true for me.
Finishing it with a friend was a gift.

On your wellness journey (or any journey in life), you will have obstacles to overcome and setbacks to recover from. You will have good days and bad days. You will feel strong and motivated and powerful one day and then the next you may feel defeated, vulnerable and hopeless. Ultimately it comes down to choices we make in life. We can stay stuck in our self-defeating stories, or we can dig deep and do what needs to be done to pull ourselves out of our self-doubt and into the light. It is our choice.

I wrote the following sometime in 2016 during a time when I was feeling down and defeated. It is a little story about the power of positive decision making.

Sleep vs. Bootcamp

"I have not been sleeping well. I have been waking up in the middle of the night every night for the last month. I lie awake for 1-2 hours, tossing and turning and my mind is racing from one thing to the next. I am exhausted most of the time and so I have skipped many exercise sessions whether it be running, bootcamp or yoga. Because I am so tired, I have also gotten lazy with my eating. My waistline is starting to expand and I can see my old "muffin top" starting to pop it's not-so-pretty head over my pants. I wonder if people are noticing. I am a bit concerned: I have lost and regained weight many times before, and for a brief moment I think that maybe this is the beginning of the end of my weight loss. But, I know how much I learned this time around, and I know that I changed some bad habits and I know a new way of eating and I know that exercise is as important as breathing, What I learned was life-changing, so I am reassured that I am not on a slippery slope to regaining my weight. I may have slipped a little, but, I will remember what I learned and I will start again. I know how to do this.

The last two nights I have slept much better and I have woken in the morning feeling more refreshed. But, I am still tired and I contemplate going back to bed so that I can continue to catch up on my sleep. As I lay there I start to think about my choices.

1. *I could go back to bed and fall back to sleep which would be great if I actually slept. However, if I did then I would miss bootcamp.*
2. *I could go back to bed and not fall back to sleep and end up tossing and turning. If this happened, I would miss bootcamp and then I would feel like crap for two reasons: no sleep and no bootcamp.*
3. *I could get up, face the day and go to bootcamp. I know from experience that if I go to bootcamp, I have a 100% chance of feeling better. I may still be tired, but I will certainly feel more energized after a good workout.*

I contemplate my three choices while lying in my warm bed. I decide to go with the sure thing that will make me feel better: I choose option #3. So, I get up, get dressed and go to bootcamp. And just as I anticipated, I felt great after my workout; it works every time! I knew I had made the right decision, and besides, I could always catch a nap later in the day!

Turning my energy level around and getting my body to bootcamp is my job. I am responsible for how I feel, and how I feel is largely due to the foods I eat and the exercise I get. Trust me, I know how it feels to have zero energy and all you want to do is sleep and shove chocolate in your face. But, learn to resist the urge to take that road, instead train yourself and your brain to take a new road. Choose to get out of bed, or off the couch; choose movement and real food that supplies life-giving energy and vitality. It feels great and it works every time."

The struggle is real and I have felt it many, many times. I wrote this poem one afternoon as I struggled to get my butt out the door and go for my run. I made a choice and it paid off.

Motivation for Running (or Life)
I really didn't feel like running,
But I got dressed anyway.
Then I looked like a runner.
Then I felt like a runner.
Then I did what runners do,
I went for a run.
And now I feel better.

What are those old sayings? *"Get up, dress up, show up." "Fake it until you make it."* Never stop believing in a better way. Never stop believing in health and well-being for you and your family. Do what needs to be done and never quit. The choice is yours. What are you going to choose?

Realize that setbacks, obstacles, and disappointment are all part of the journey of life. No one gets out without some bruises, cuts, scrapes and scars. But, don't let these misfortunes define who you are. Sometimes the best lessons and opportunities are born from the worst experiences. When you get struck down, get back up, dust yourself off, lick your wounds if you must, but put a smile on your face and keep moving forwards .

Remember, sometimes we need to rest, and sometimes we need to look obstacles in the face and say:

"Not this time, this time I call the shots,
this time I am stronger than you!"

Chapter 12

The Road to Health and Wellness

As I near the end of my book I am filled with so much gratitude for the things that I have learned, for the inspiration to put my words on paper, and for the people who have helped me and believed in me along the way.

When I first started to write down my story I had no idea how it was going to unfold and what the final book would look like. Many of my original writings are not even part of this story. The book grew and developed as I continued to write down my thoughts. Some of my thoughts came in the middle of the night, or as I was running, or driving or just out doing errands. Some of my thoughts were forced as I sat at my desk not knowing what to write or how to write it. But, I persevered. I often started these forced writing sessions by saying: *"I don't know what to write today, I don't really have anything inspirational coming to me, so I guess I will just write about….."* Then sure enough, the words would start coming to me and I would usually end those writing sessions with something that I could use. Eventually, I had enough material that I could start sorting it into chapter ideas. Again, I still had no idea what the final product would look like but I kept moving forward.

One summer day several months into my journey I was outside washing out our garbage cans. I was thinking about my book and then suddenly as clear as could be I heard a voice inside me say, **"If you write it, you will be supported."**

These clear and precise words became instrumental in my journey. When I was feeling stuck, full of doubt, unsure of my message or frustrated with the progress of my writing, I would come back to these words that were spoken to me that summer day: *"If you write it, you will be supported."* So, I continued to write, change, and re-write until I had what I thought to be a pretty decent account of the steps I took on my journey to reclaim my health.

My dream was that by sharing my story perhaps I would be able to inspire a few people to look at their own health and lifestyle choices; maybe find some inspiration or motivation to make some positive changes that would improve the quality of their lives.

My dream and those inspirational words kept me going.

Once my manuscript was ready for another set of eyes I asked a few people to read it over and give me their opinion. One of those people was my brother David. A few days after I had given him a copy I received a text from him:

D: A quick question:
- *Does a healthy person eat pie?*

Me: Lol! Good question. Something to ponder.... I think a healthy person would enjoy one piece of pie....unhealthy people eat more than one piece... (as I point a finger at my old self).

A few weeks later we talked on the phone and he informed me that he bought himself a tricycle. I thought that was very cool. I asked him what made him decide to buy a tricycle and he said to me: "Because that's what healthy people do!"

My heart swells a little!

Mother's Day 2018 rolls around and as usual I get to do whatever I want to do that day. I decide I want to go visit my brother and his partner Liane and go for a bike ride. So, that's what we did. My heart was filled with so much joy at watching my brother ride his tricycle as happily and joyfully as a five year old. His grin was from ear to ear and he exuded happiness. This is what a healthy lifestyle is all about.

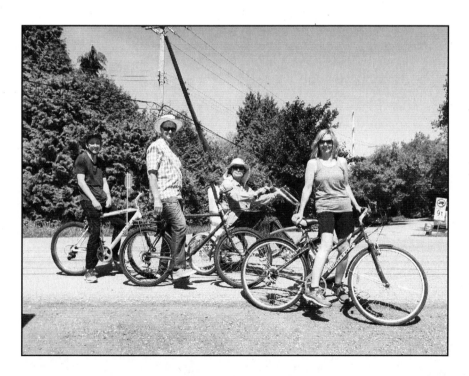

Mother's Day 2018 with my son, husband and brother.

A couple of more weeks go by and I received another text from my brother. It was a picture of a delicious looking meal with the following text:

D: Breakfast, Kale, onion & egg
   pizza crust with on-the-vine
   tomatoes, marble & feta
   cheeses, basil and ranch
   dressing.

Me: Did you make this?
   It looks amazing and
   sounds delicious.

D: Yep. I did it. It is what
   a healthy person eats, LOL...

Me: I love it!

And I really do love it. I love that my manuscript inspired my brother to question whether he should buy a pie. I love that he was inspired to purchase a tricycle, and I love that he was inspired to make such a delicious, healthy breakfast and then to share the picture with me all in the name of doing what healthy people do. It makes my heart really, really happy.

You see, my brother has been fighting his own battle since January 2015 when he was diagnosed with leukemia. He ended up receiving a bone marrow transplant from my sister Dianne. He had several rounds of chemotherapy and radiation. He has been through multiple other procedures in dealing with the effects of graft vs host disease which for him means he has developed a skin condition that makes his skin ultra-sensitive, itchy and scaly. But, through all his treatment, he has stayed positive and began his own quest to improve his health. He did lots of research on healthy eating and joined an organization in Vancouver called *"Inspired Health"* where he could take classes on nutrition and learn more about how to heal his body using food as important and life-giving *"medicine."*

His journey has been nothing short of life-changing.

In an earlier chapter I talked about my experience of running the 2017 **Vancouver BMO Marathon** and I mentioned that although the runner in me was disappointed with my finish time, that I wouldn't have traded some of the experiences for anything. Three of those experiences had to do with my brother because along the course I saw him and Liane not once, not twice, but three times. These moments were precious and so unexpected. The fact that he was able to make it out to cheer me on was so great. Then I saw him again a few kilometers later and my heart was so excited. He even had energy to run with me for a hundred meters or so. This experience was so joyful. Then he and Liane, along with my husband, son and brother-in-law were all at the finish line. This was so amazing because my brother was there! He was alive and he was out experiencing life and *cheering me on*! What a wonderful gift!

I share these stories of my brother because when I see him changing what he eats, and riding his bicycle and cheering me on during a race, I know that he is making a choice to identify as a healthy person. He has not let cancer define him. In fact, it's almost the opposite. He was given a very challenging experience in life, but, he is choosing healthy! He is choosing to do what healthy people do and his choices are paying off as he continues to get stronger, healthier and happier.

Being fit and strong and healthy is not an automatic for most people. Some people's roads to wellness will be longer and bumpier. Some people will find smoother paths. Each of us will have our own path to follow.

Health and wellness is not just for a few specially selected people, it is available to everyone. But, you need to take control, ask questions, listen, and then experiment with different ways of doing things. You will need to be open to change and make positive decisions one step at a time. That's what I did and as a result I lost 45 pounds. That's what my brother is doing and as a result he is regaining his health.

I am filled with joy that my words have inspired him to think like a healthy person, and I want the same for you.

When I look around, I see a lot of people suffering and it makes me sad because it doesn't have to stay that way. Life will change when you do. Choose health and watch as the seeds of wellness sprout and grow.

So, in closing, I would like to leave you with this one final thought:

What would a healthy person do?

Then go do that!

In health and wellness,
Love
Rhonda
eat • breathe • grow

Recipes

Breakfast

Soups and Salads

Pizza and Pasta

Treats and Desserts

Breakfast

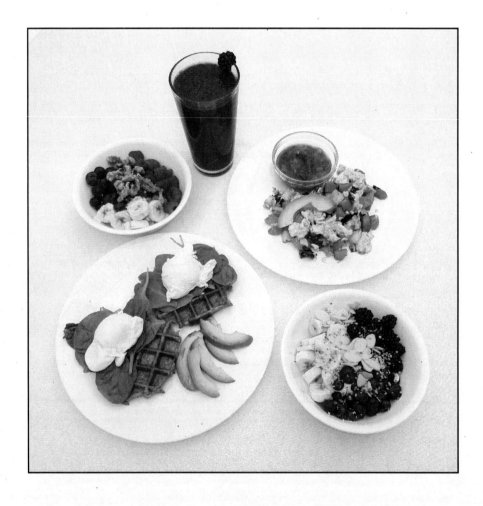

Pretty in Pink Frozen Goodness – by Rhonda
Wheat-free, Dairy-free, Serves 2 - 4

1 cup of coconut water
1 cup of orange juice
1 cup frozen spinach or kale
½ cup frozen beets
¼ of a long English cucumber
1 banana
½ cup frozen peaches or berries
1 scoop of protein powder (optional)

1. Put all ingredients in a blender and blend until well mixed and smooth.
2. Pour into a bowl or glass.
3. Grab a spoon and enjoy, but, don't eat too fast, you will get brain-freeze!

Scrambled eggs with vegetables
Wheat-free, Dairy-free, 1 to 2 servings

1. Whisk 2 eggs together.
2. Add 1 – 2 tbsp of oil to a hot pan.
3. Quickly stir-fry whatever vegetables you have on hand.
4. Add eggs, stir until cooked.
5. Serve egg dish with a side of salsa and avocado.

Yam Waffles - by Rhonda
Wheat-free, Dairy-free, makes approximately 6 waffles

2 cups of grated yams – pat any excess moisture out with a paper towel
2 eggs
1 tbsp chia seeds or flax seeds
2 tbsp coconut flour
1 tbsp maple syrup
1 tsp cinnamon
½ tsp salt

1. Mix all ingredients together.
2. Let rest for 5-10 minutes.
3. Brush waffle iron with coconut oil.
4. Scoop approximately ¼ cup of mixture into each waffle section.
5. Cook until crispy, about 5 minutes – steam will rise as it cooks so be careful when opening lid.
6. Carefully remove waffles then top with spinach, poached or basted eggs, avocado and a drizzle of maple syrup.

Oatmeal with fruit and nuts
Wheat-free, dairy-free

1. Cook old-fashioned oats according to the directions on the package.
2. Add desired fruit part way through the cooking process. (Note that apples will take longer to cook and some fruit just needs to be warmed if at all.)
3. Remove from heat and pour oatmeal into a bowl.
4. Top with more fruit if desired as well as nuts and/or seeds of your choice.
5. Add a splash of almond milk and a bit of sweetener as desired. I use maple syrup or a teaspoon of jam.

Greek Yogurt with fruit and seeds
Wheat Free

1. Scoop a serving of Greek yogurt into a bowl.
2. Add sliced fruit to yogurt.
3. Top with nuts or seeds of your choice.
4. Add a dash of maple syrup, jam or honey to taste.

Soups and Salads

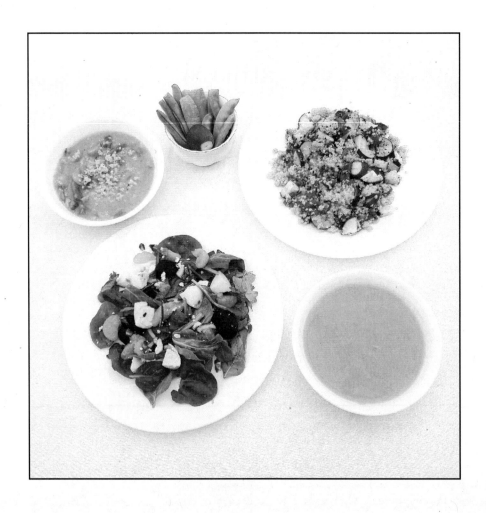

Simple Delicious Homemade Soup – by Rhonda

1. Sauté 1 onion and 2-3 cloves of garlic in 2 tbsp of oil (olive oil, grapeseed oil, avocado oil, coconut oil or butter)

2. Add 3-4 cups of chopped vegetables of your choice, stir for 1-2 minutes
    -   broccoli & cauliflower
    -   carrots & squash
    -   asparagus & celery
    -   potatoes & broccoli
    -   potatoes & leeks
    -   mushrooms
    -   tomatoes (I blanch the tomatoes first to remove the skins. I also cut them up and remove the seeds before adding them to the soup mixture.)

3. Add 4-6 cups of liquid
    -   chicken stock
    -   vegetable stock
    -   water
    -   coconut milk (goes great with carrots, yams and squash based soups)
    -   or a combination of 2 or more liquids

4. Cover and let simmer for 20-30 minutes until vegetables are soft

5. Add salt, pepper, herbs and spices.
    - cumin and ginger go good with squash and carrots
    - rosemary goes good with mushrooms
    - curry powder pairs well with cauliflower
    - basil and thyme are perfect in tomato soup
    - thyme also works well in potato soup.

6. Simmer for another 10 minutes and then remove from heat and let cool a bit.
    - I like to blend my soups using a hand-held immersion blender but you can also pour the soup into a blender (be careful that the soup isn't too hot as the hot soup might explode in the blender).
    - You can blend it up completely, or leave some of it unblended to add extra texture to your soup.
    - I often add cooked quinoa, chicken chunks and previously cooked vegetables to my soup to make it more like chowder.

7. Enjoy your homemade soup knowing that it is delicious and nutritious and will fuel your body with warmth and energy.

Shawna's Sensational Spinach Salad – by Shawna Stonehouse-Lawson
Wheat-free

Spinach
Cooked beets – cubed
Hard-boiled egg – sliced
Candied pecans (I usually use roasted pecans)
Mandarin orange sections (I have also used chopped dates)
Feta cheese
Thinly sliced red onion

Dressing:
3 parts poppy seed dressing (I have also used ranch or Caesar salad dressing)
1 part orange juice concentrate

1. Mix salad ingredients in large bowl using whatever quantities you like.
2. In a small bowl whisk the orange juice concentrate with the dressing.
3. Pour dressing over salad.
4. Serve and enjoy.

The Accidental Quinoa Vegetable Salad – by Rhonda
Wheat-free, dairy-free, makes 2-4 servings

1 cup of cooked quinoa
½ cup chopped roasted red and/or yellow peppers
1/3 of an English cucumber - chopped
2 or 3 thinly sliced radishes
½ of a diced avocado
2 tbsp of olive oil
A squeeze of lemon or lime juice
A sprinkle of Italian seasoning
A dash of salt and pepper

1. Mix all ingredients together and serve.
2. Salad keeps well in the fridge for a day or two.

Pizza and Pasta

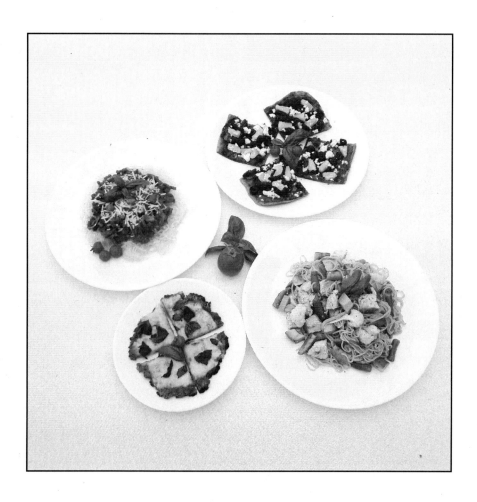

Cauliflower Quinoa Crusts – By Rhonda
Wheat-free, makes six - 6" round crusts

1 medium head of cauliflower – cut into bites size pieces
1 cup of cooked quinoa
¾ cup of shredded cheese (your choice)
¼ cup of chopped parsley, basil or chives
2 eggs
2 tbsp of chia seeds
2 tbsp of coconut flour
2 tsp of chopped garlic
Salt and pepper

1. Preheat oven to 375 degrees.
2. Toss cauliflower in olive oil then spread out on baking sheet.
3. Roast cauliflower for about 25 minutes until golden brown.
4. Remove from oven and let cauliflower cool. (You can roast this in advance.)
5. In a food processor add the cauliflower and all the remaining ingredients. Mix until well blended.
6. Line 2 baking sheets with parchment paper.
7. Divide mixture into 6 equal balls. Place each ball on the baking sheet and flatten. Each crust will be about 6" in diameter.
8. Increase oven temperature to 425 degrees.
9. Bake the crusts for about 15 minutes.
10. Remove from oven, let cool for a few minutes, then carefully move each crust onto a cooling rack.
11. You can then proceed to make a pizza or grilled cheese sandwich.

12. To make grilled cheese, simply add whatever cheese you like between 2 layers of crust and grill in a hot oiled pan. Flip to brown both sides.

13. If you freeze the crusts, make sure to put parchment paper between each crust so they don't stick together.

Family Favourite Quinoa Pizza Crust – by Rhonda (inspired by simplyquinoa.com)
Wheat-free, Dairy-free crusts, makes two 10' round or rectangle crusts

1 cup of quinoa (soaked in water for 6-8 hours)
1/3 cup of water
1 tsp Italian seasoning
3/4 tsp baking powder
½ tsp. garlic powder
1/2 tsp salt
2 tbsp olive oil (divided)

1. Preheat oven to 425 degrees.
2. Line a rectangular baking sheet with parchment paper. Drizzle paper with 1 tbsp of olive oil and spread it around with your hands to evenly coat the paper. (If you are going to make 3 crusts, you will probably need to prepare 2 baking sheets with parchment paper and oil.)
3. Rinse the soaked quinoa and add to blender.
4. Add 1/3 cup of water, Italian seasoning, baking powder, garlic powder, salt and remaining 1 tbsp of olive oil.
5. Blend on high speed until the batter resembles a thick batter.

6. Pour the batter into the prepared pans and spread evenly. (I usually pour the batter into two or three smaller pizza crusts.) Bake for 10 minutes. Remove, flip the crusts and continue baking for another 10 minutes.

7. Remove from oven. You can continue to make your pizza by adding sauce and toppings as desired, bake for another 10-15 minutes. Or, you can let the crusts cool and save them for use at another time. These crusts freeze well and are easy to defrost.

Spaghetti Squash and Your Choice Sauce

Wheat-free, to make Dairy-free eliminate the cheese
One spaghetti squash makes 4-6 servings.

One spaghetti squash
Meat sauce or tomato sauce of your choice
Diced vegetables of your choice
Sprinkle of parmesan cheese
chili flakes and salt and pepper as desired

1. Cut spaghetti squash in half lengthwise and remove the seeds.

2. Rub squash with olive oil, place faced down on baking sheet and roast in 375 degree oven for 45-50 minutes (or until squash is tender crisp).

3. Meanwhile, make your favourite meat or vegetable sauce. I like to add lots of extra vegetables to my meat sauce. I dice up carrots and peppers add mushrooms, chopped broccoli, spinach or grated zucchini.

4. Once squash is cooked remove from oven and let cool enough

so that you can handle it. Cut or peel away the outer shell, then shred the spaghetti squash with a fork or you can pull apart with your hands. (You can use squash immediately or refrigerate to use another day. It also freezes well.)

5. On a plate layer the spaghetti squash, meat and vegetable sauce and sprinkle with a bit of parmesan cheese, chili flakes, and salt and pepper.

Ramen Noodles Using Leftover Vegetables and Chicken
Wheat-free

Ramen noodles (made from organic millet and brown rice), 1 ramen cake per person
Precooked vegetables of your choice
Precooked chicken (or seafood)
Pesto – approximately 1-2 tbsp per serving
½-1 diced avocado
Parmesan cheese
Salt and pepper

1. Select whatever leftover vegetables you have on hand. I use carrots, cauliflower, broccoli, green beans, asparagus, peppers, or whatever is in my fridge. (If you don't have any, cook some up by steaming them or roasting them.)
2. Chop up leftover chicken or seafood. (If you don't have any cook some up.)
3. Once the chicken and vegetables are ready, cook the ramen noodles as per directions on package.

4. Drain and rinse the noodles.

5. Return the noodles to the pot then add pesto, the diced avocado, the cooked vegetables and the cooked chicken. Mix together.

6. Leave the pot on low for a few minutes to warm the vegetables and chicken or seafood.

7. Sprinkle with parmesan cheese, and salt and pepper as desired. Serve.

Treats and Desserts

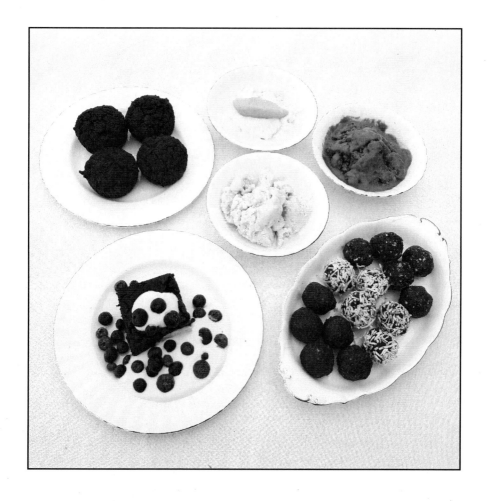

Chocolate Zucchini Quinoa Muffins – by Rhonda
Wheat-free, Dairy-free, makes 12 muffins

Wet Ingredients:
1 ½ cups of grated zucchini
1 cup of cooked quinoa
½ cup of almond milk
¼ cup of maple syrup
1 tsp. of vanilla

Dry Ingredients:
½ cup of finely ground oats (gluten-free if available)
½ cup of buckwheat flour
½ cup of cocoa powder
⅓ cup coconut palm or cane sugar
1 tbsp flax seeds
1 tsp baking powder
½ tsp baking soda
½ tsp salt

Add at end:
2 tbsp of melted coconut oil
¼ cup mini dark chocolate chips

1. Preheat oven to 350 degrees.
2. Grate the zucchini by hand or use your food processor grating blade.
3. Switch blade in food processor to mixing blade, then add all remaining wet ingredients into the zucchini, process until well combined.

4. In a medium bowl mix together all dry ingredients.
5. Add dry ingredients to the food processor and mix everything together.
6. Stir in the coconut oil and ¼ cup of mini dark chocolate chips.
7. Line muffin tins with parchment paper cups and equally divide the batter into 12 muffins.
8. Bake at 350 degrees for 20 minutes.
9. Remove from oven and let cool for about 10 minutes before removing from muffin tins. Let cool completely before storing
10. Muffins will keep in fridge for several days. They also freeze well.

Black Bean and Avocado Chocolate Brownie – by Rhonda
Wheat-free, Dairy-free

Wet ingredients:
1 can of rinsed and drained organic black beans
3 eggs
1 small ripe avocado (or ½ of a large avocado)
½ cup of maple syrup
½ cup almond milk
2 tsp. vanilla

Dry ingredients:
½ cup good quality cocoa powder
⅓ cup ground flax seeds
⅓ cup coconut palm sugar
¼ cup buckwheat flour

1 tsp baking powder

1 tsp baking soda

½ tsp salt

Optional:

¼ cup mini dark chocolate chips + 2 tbsp to sprinkle on top

1. Preheat oven to 350 degrees.
2. Line a 9" x 9" round or square cake pan with parchment paper.
3. In a blender add all the wet ingredients. Blend until batter is smooth and creamy looking. Pour batter into a large mixing bowl.
4. In a small bowl combine the dry ingredients.
5. Slowly pour the dry ingredients into the wet batter. Mix well.
6. Add chocolate chips to batter (if using them).
7. Pour batter into prepared cake pan.
8. Sprinkle the 2 tbsp of chocolate chips on top (if you are using them).
9. Bake at 350 degrees for 40-45 minutes or until a toothpick comes out clean when inserted into the center of the brownie.
10. Let cake pan rest for 10 minutes before carefully lifting the brownie out of the pan by gently pulling up on the sides of the parchment paper.
11. Cool completely and then refrigerate.
12. Brownie is best served cold with creamy topping recipe below.
13. To make it extra special, top with some fresh organic berries.

Creamy Topping - by Rhonda

½ cup of Greek yogurt

½ cup of sour cream

1 tbsp of orange juice or mango concentrate

1 tbsp of maple syrup

1. Mix all ingredients together and serve on top or on the side of the chocolate brownie.
2. Top with fresh berries as desired.

Almond Date Dark Cacao Balls – By Patti Fleury

Wheat-free, dairy-free, makes about 14-16 one-inch balls

1 ½ cups of dates (if using dry dates soak for 2 hours)

1 cup of finely ground almonds

3 tbsp raw cacao (or good quality cocoa)

1 tbsp almond butter

1 tbsp coconut oil

2 tsp cinnamon

Shredded coconut (optional)

Version #2 – I add these ingredients when I am making these balls to take with me on my long runs.

Add ½ cup of oatmeal

2 tbsp of honey

1 tsp salt

1. Blend all ingredients in food processor (except shredded coconut).
2. Roll into balls.
3. Roll in shredded coconut if desired.
4. Refrigerate.

Peach Ice Dream – by Rhonda

Makes 2-4 servings

1 cup of plain Greek yogurt
1 cup of frozen peaches
¼ cup coconut milk
2 tbsp of peach juice
1 tsp of vanilla
1- 2 tbsp of maple syrup or organic cane sugar (depending on how sweet your peaches are)

1. Put all ingredients into a blender and mix until smooth and creamy.
2. Adjust sweetness as desired.
3. Pour into a bowl and enjoy.

Coconut Banana Ice Dream – by Rhonda

Makes 4-8 servings

1 – 400ml can of organic coconut milk
1 cup of almond milk
1 very ripe banana

¼ cup of maple syrup

½ tsp vanilla

1. Add all ingredients to a blender, mix until smooth.
2. Pour into a freezer-proof bowl and put it into the freezer.
3. Stir every ½ hour until almost frozen. (If you let it freeze solid you will have to let it thaw out for a bit before serving it.)
4. Scoop into bowl and enjoy.

Chocolate Coconut Banana Ice Dream – by Rhonda

Makes 4-8 servings

Same as above except add:

¼ cup of good quality cocoa and 2 more tbsp of maple syrup to the blender.

Author Biography

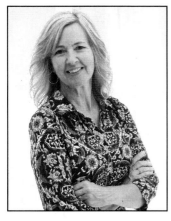

Rhonda was put on her first diet when she was just 11 years old. That diet started a rollercoaster ride of weight loss and weight gain for almost 40 years. At the age of 50, Rhonda's life took an abrupt and unexpected turn that made her stop and take a good look in the mirror. What she saw was a very unhealthy, overweight, and unhappy person. She knew she had to do something or her health would only continue to decline. But, going on another failed diet was not the solution. Instead, she began a journey to reclaim her health by making one healthy decision at a time. In this book, Rhonda shares her story of how she stopped dieting, lost 45 pounds and rediscovered a whole new side of food and fitness.

Rhonda is now living the active, outgoing, healthy lifestyle that she only ever dreamt of. She loves to share healthy, delicious meals with her friends and family. She is an avid runner and has completed two marathons. In the summer months, Rhonda grows a variety of fruits and vegetables in her backyard garden. She lives in Abbotsford, Canada with her husband, son, and dog Elly-May.

You can see more of Rhonda's Eat Breathe Grow Lifestyle on her social media accounts:

Instagram: @eatbreathegrow
Facebook: Eat Breathe Grow with Rhonda
Website: eatbreathegrow.com